WITHDRAWN

Whittle's Gait Analysis
Fifth Edition

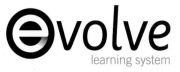

learning system

Evolve Learning Resources for Students and Lecturers.

Access to the website: http://evolve.elsevier.com/Whittle/gait

Think outside the book... evolve

For Elsevier
Commissioning Editor: Rita Demetriou-Swanwick
Development Editor: Nicola Lally
Project Manager: Sruthi Viswam
Designer/Design Direction: Stewart Larking
Illustration Manager: Merlyn Harvey/Jennifer Rose

Whittle's Gait Analysis

Fifth Edition

Edited by

David Levine PT PhD DPT OCS

Professor and Walter M. Cline Chair of Excellence, The University of Tennessee at Chattanooga, Chattanooga, Tennessee, USA

Jim Richards BEng MSc PhD

Professor of Biomechanics & Research Lead for Allied Health; School of Sport, Tourism & the Outdoors, University of Central Lancashire, UK

Michael W. Whittle BSc MSc MB BS PhD

Formerly Walter M. Cline Jr Chair of Rehabilitation Technology, The University of Tennessee at Chattanooga, Chattanooga, Tennessee, USA; Director, H. Carey Hanlin Motion Analysis Laboratory, The University of Tennessee at Chattanooga, Chattanooga, TN, USA; Formerly Acting Director, Oxford Orthopaedic Engineering Centre, University of Oxford, Oxford, UK

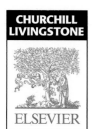

CHURCHILL LIVINGSTONE

ELSEVIER

Edinburgh   London   New York   Oxford   Philadelphia   St Louis   Sydney   Toronto   2012

CHURCHILL
LIVINGSTONE
ELSEVIER

First edition 1990
Second edition 1996
Third edition 2002
Fourth edition 2007
Fifth edition 2012
   Reprinted 2013 (twice), 2014 (twice)

ISBN 978-0-7020-4265-2

British Library Cataloguing in Publication Data
A catalogue record for this book is available from the British Library

Library of Congress Cataloging in Publication Data
A catalog record for this book is available from the Library of Congress

Notices

Knowledge and best practice in this field are constantly changing. As new research and experience broaden our understanding, changes in research methods, professional practices, or medical treatment may become necessary.

Practitioners and researchers must always rely on their own experience and knowledge in evaluating and using any information, methods, compounds, or experiments described herein. In using such information or methods they should be mindful of their own safety and the safety of others, including parties for whom they have a professional responsibility.

With respect to any drug or pharmaceutical products identified, readers are advised to check the most current information provided (i) on procedures featured or (ii) by the manufacturer of each product to be administered, to verify the recommended dose or formula, the method and duration of administration, and contraindications. It is the responsibility of practitioners, relying on their own experience and knowledge of their patients, to make diagnoses, to determine dosages and the best treatment for each individual patient, and to take all appropriate safety precautions.

To the fullest extent of the law, neither the Publisher nor the authors, contributors, or editors, assume any liability for any injury and/or damage to persons or property as a matter of products liability, negligence or otherwise, or from any use or operation of any methods, products, instructions, or ideas contained in the material herein.

ELSEVIER your source for books,
journals and multimedia
in the health sciences
www.elsevierhealth.com

Working together to grow
libraries in developing countries

www.elsevier.com | www.bookaid.org | www.sabre.org

ELSEVIER BOOK AID International Sabre Foundation

The
Publisher's
policy is to use
**paper manufactured
from sustainable forests**

Printed in China

Last digit is the print number: 9 8 7 6 5

Contents

Evolve Resources (web contents)

The additional online resources can be found on our Evolve learning system.

For access please go to http://evolve.elsevier.com/Whittle/gait and follow the onscreen prompts. Contents include:

- Video clips
- Image collection from the book
- MCQs
- Appendix 1 – Conversions between measurement units
- Appendix 2 – Contributors to Whittle's Gait Analysis, Fifth Edition
- Glossary

Acknowledgements

Many thanks are owed when a book several years in the formation is finally completed. So many people have generously given their time and thoughts to help me, that they cannot all be listed; however, a few special people should be thanked by name for their support and encouragement. Gratitude to my co-editors and friends, Jim Richards and of course the person after whom this book is named, Mike Whittle. They are not only exceptional teachers, researchers, and writers but exceptional people. I also would like to thank the many contributors who have helped to keep this work spirited and always enjoyable. My colleagues, students, and patients, I continue to learn everyday from all of you. Old friends, like Kevin, Ivan, Denis, Darryl, and Randy who have kept me laughing for the last 25 plus years, let's keep the good times coming! To many family members across this country who remind me of what family means, and to the memory of my father, Jacob Levine (1913-2011). To my mother Marie, to whom I owe much more than I can ever repay. Because of my parents I grew up realizing that living life according to the Golden Rule was the only way to live. Their strong work ethic and loyalty have been indispensable life lessons. My children Lauren, Sarah, Hadley, and Ava who make every day a new adventure and share it with me. My best friend Allison who understands me completely and supports me wholly. And to the one who was with me before I was born.

David Levine

I wish to thank Michael Whittle who has intrusted the 5th edition of his excellent book to us and I sincerely hope that he is as pleased with the result as we are. Thanks also to David Levine and to all the contributors for their tireless work and contributions. I also owe an enormous debt of gratitude to all my colleagues and students past and present, who I have learned so much from. Thanks, as ever, to my wife Jackie for her support and to my children Imogen and Joe who keep me grounded.

Jim Richards

Preface

Gait analysis is the systematic study of human walking, using the eye and brain of experienced observers, augmented by instrumentation for measuring body movements, body mechanics and the activity of the muscles. In individuals with conditions affecting their ability to walk, gait analysis may be used to make detailed diagnoses and to plan optimal treatment.

The first four editions of this book have made a significant contribution to the use of Gait Analysis worldwide, supported by the fact that the current editors and contributors were all influenced by Professor Michael Whittle's earlier editions. We hope this latest edition, as with the previous editions, provides a text which does not require a high level of academic learning to be understood, but yet gives a good grounding in the science and application of gait analysis. In this edition we have added the contributions of several clinicians who are experts in their respective areas of gait analysis.

Over the last decade, gait analysis has "come of age" and many clinicians now use it routinely to provide the best possible care for many groups of patients. This is most notable within the management of cerebral palsy, however gait analysis is beginning to be used more widely within other neurological and musculoskeletal conditions. For this reason, two additional chapters have been added to this textbook: "Gait assessment in neurological disorders", and "Gait analysis in musculoskeletal conditions, prosthetics and orthotics". Since the advantages of this approach have been well established, it is to be hoped that its usage will continue to spread, so that many more will benefit from the treatment decisions which can be made when gait analysis is used.

Improvements in the ease and speed with which gait data can be collected and interpreted, coupled with decreases in the cost of the equipment and the skill level needed to use it have led to significant strides in gait analysis since the fourth edition of the book. This edition aims to show the current uses of gait analysis and guidance on how it can be applied to wider groups of patients. We have also included examples of new and evolving methods of analysis which may in the future further improve the levels of analysis we can currently achieve. The book is targeted at physicians, physiotherapists, prosthetists, orthotists, podiatrists, and anyone interested in human gait analysis.

We have also included examples of 'real' gait data of a variety of clinical case studies which we hope will provide the reader with a greater opportunity to get a feel for this fascinating subject and its clinical impact. We are honored to have been appointed editors of this textbook.

Jim Richards and David Levine, 2012

Biography of Dr Michael Whittle

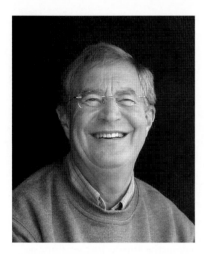

Michael Whittle, was the sole author and editor of the first four editions of this textbook. Although a medical doctor, Mike was destined to become a research scientist with degrees in biomechanics and a Ph.D. in human biology and health from the University of Surrey. As an exchange medical officer in the Royal Air Force, he was loaned to NASA to supervise six of the medical experiments on the Skylab space program in the 1970's. He later joined the faculty of the University of Oxford, and carried out pioneering work on the scientific measurement of gait analysis. Mike moved to the University of Tennessee at Chattanooga in 1989 and was a professor in the Department of Physical Therapy, and also in the Department of Orthopaedic Surgery of the University of Tennessee College of Medicine. He continued his research on gait analysis and established the H. Carey Hanlin motion analysis laboratory which was one of the first motion analysis laboratories of its kind. Having had the privilege of working with Mike on a daily basis for 15 years (DL), he is an exceptional researcher, teacher, and scientist whose greatest asset is an inquisitive mind with a delightful personality to match it.

Now retired to the South of England, he enjoys travelling, sailing, hiking, and spending time with his wife Wendy, their children, and grandchildren. In his honour this book has been renamed Whittle's Gait Analysis.

Contributors

Julie Bage PT DPT OCS
Adjunct Faculty, University of Tennessee at Chattanooga,
Department of Physical Therapy, Chattanooga,
Tennessee, USA

Richard Baker PhD CEng CSci
Professor of Clinical Gait Analysis, University of Salford,
Salford, UK

Gabor Barton Dr MD
Reader in Biomechanics, Research Institute for Sport and
Exercise Sciences, Liverpool John Moores University,
Liverpool, UK

Douglas Daniel DPT
Physical Therapist, Patrick Rehab-Wellness Center,
Fayetteville, Tennessee, USA

Nancy Fell PhD PT NCS
Associate Professor, Department of Physical Therapy
and University of Tennessee at Chattanooga,
Chattanooga, Tennessee, USA

David Levine PT PhD DPT OCS
Professor and Walter M. Cline Chair
of Excellence, The University of Tennessee
at Chattanooga, Chattanooga, Tennessee, USA

Jim Richards BEng MSc PhD
Professor of Biomechanics & Research Lead for Allied
Health; School of Sport, Tourism & the Outdoors,
University of Central Lancashire, UK

Cathie Smith PhD DPT PCS
Associate Professor, Department of Physical Therapy,
University of Tennessee at Chattanooga, Chattanooga,
Tennessee, USA

Jeremiah Tate PhD PT
Assistant Professor, Department of Physical Therapy,
University of Tennessee at Chattanooga, Chattanooga,
Tennessee, USA

Natalie Vanicek PhD
Senior Lecturer in Clinical Biomechanics, Exercise and
Sport Science, Faculty of Health Sciences, The University
of Sydney, Australia

Basic sciences

1

Michael Whittle   David Levine   Jim Richards

All voluntary movement, including walking, results from a complicated process involving the brain, spinal cord, peripheral nerves, muscles, bones and joints. Before considering in detail the process of walking, what can go wrong with it and how it can be studied, it is necessary to have a basic understanding of three scientific disciplines: anatomy, physiology and biomechanics. It is hoped that this chapter will provide the rudiments of these subjects for those not already familiar with them, review the topic for those who are, and also provide a convenient source of reference material.

Anatomy

It is not the intention of this book to teach in detail the anatomy of the locomotor system, which is well covered in several other books (e.g. *Gray's Anatomy*, 2009). The notes which follow give only an outline of the subject, but one which should be sufficient for an understanding of gait analysis. The anatomical names for the different parts of the body vary somewhat from one textbook to another, and as far as possible the most common name has been used. The section starts by describing some basic anatomical terms and then goes on to describe the bones, joints, muscles and nervous system. Although the arteries and veins are essential to the functioning of the locomotor system, they will not be described here since they generally affect gait only indirectly, through their role in providing oxygen and nutrients for the nerves and muscles and removing waste products.

Basic anatomical terms

The anatomical terms describing the relationships between different parts of the body are based on the *anatomical position*, in which a person is standing upright, with the feet together and the arms by the sides of the body, with the palms forward. This position, together with the reference planes and the terms describing the relationships between different parts of the body, is illustrated in Figure 1.1.

Six terms are used to describe directions in relation to the centre of the body. These are best defined by example:

1. The umbilicus is *anterior*
2. The buttocks are *posterior*
3. The head is *superior*
4. The feet are *inferior*
5. *Left* is self-evident
6. So is *right*.

The anterior surface of the body is *ventral* and the posterior surface is *dorsal*. The word *dorsum* is used for both the back of the hand and the upper surface of the foot. The terms *cephal* (towards the head) and *caudal* (towards the 'tail') are sometimes used in place of superior and inferior.

Within a single part of the body, six additional terms are used to describe relationships:

1. *Medial* means towards the midline of the body: the big toe is on the medial side of the foot
2. *Lateral* means away from the midline of the body: the little toe is on the lateral side of the foot
3. *Proximal* means towards the rest of the body: the shoulder is the proximal part of the arm

The motion of the limbs is described using reference planes:

1. A *sagittal* plane is any plane which divides the body into right and left portions; the *median* plane is the midline sagittal plane, which divides the whole body into right and left halves
2. A *coronal* (or *frontal*) plane divides a body part into front and back portions
3. A *transverse* (or *horizontal*) plane divides a body part into upper and lower portions.

The term *coronal plane* is equivalent to frontal plane and the transverse plane may also be called the *horizontal plane*, although it is only horizontal when in the standing position.

Most joints have their largest amount of movement in the sagittal plane, although the coronal and transverse planes can be very important clinically. The directions of these motions for the hip and knee are shown in Figure 1.2 and for the ankle and foot in Figure 1.3. The possible movements are as follows:

1. *Flexion* and *extension* take place in the sagittal plane; in the ankle these movements are called *dorsiflexion* and *plantarflexion*, where the foot (distal segment) moves up or down relative to the tibia (proximal segment), respectively
2. *Abduction* and *adduction* take place in the frontal plane, where the distal segment moves away or towards the midline of the body relative to the proximal segment, respectively

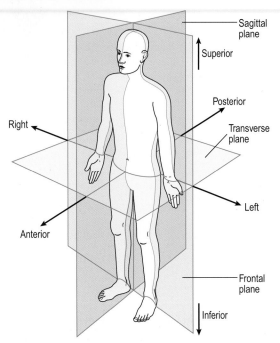

Fig. 1.1 • The anatomical position, with the three reference planes and six fundamental directions.

4. *Distal* means away from the rest of the body: the fingers are the distal part of the arm
5. *Superficial* structures are close to the surface: the skin is superficial to the bones
6. *Deep* structures are far from the surface: the heart is deep to the sternum.

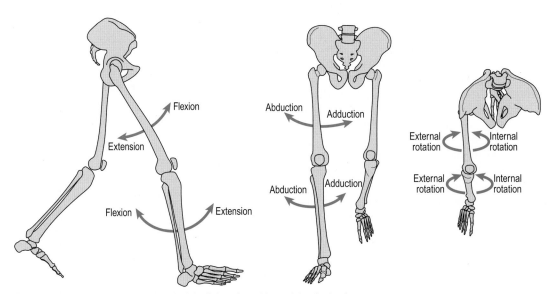

Fig. 1.2 • Movements about the hip joint (above) and knee joint (below).

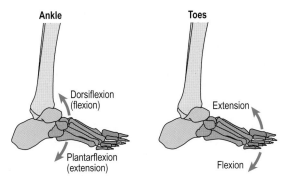

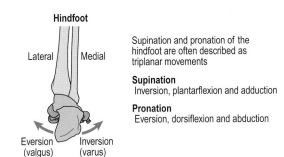

Supination and pronation of the hindfoot are often described as triplanar movements

Supination
Inversion, plantarflexion and adduction

Pronation
Eversion, dorsiflexion and abduction

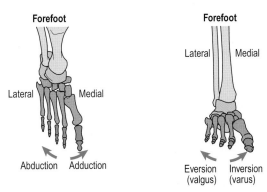

Fig. 1.3 • Movements of the ankle, toes, hindfoot and forefoot.

3. *Internal* and external rotation take place in the transverse plane; they are also called *medial* and *lateral* rotation, respectively, the term referring to the motion of the anterior surface of the distal segment relative to the proximal.

Other terms which are used to describe the motions of the joints or body segments are:

1. *Varus* (adducted) and *valgus* (abducted), which describe an angulation of a joint towards or away from the midline, respectively, when viewed in the coronal plane. Therefore knock knees are in valgus and bow legs are in varus.

2. *Pronation* and *supination*, which are internal and external rotations of the hand about the long axis of the forearm. Pronation of both hands brings the thumbs together, supination brings the little fingers together (aide memoire: you can hold soup in your hands if the palms are upwards). Internal and external rotation of the foot about the long axis of the tibia has also been used to describe pronation and supination of the foot and ankle complex.

3. *Inversion* (adduction) of the feet brings the soles together; *eversion* (abduction) causes the soles to point away from the midline when viewed in the coronal plane.

Terminology in the foot is often confusing and lacking in standardisation. This book has adopted what is probably the commonest convention (Fig. 1.3), in which the term *pronation* is used for a combined movement which consists primarily of eversion but also includes some dorsiflexion and forefoot abduction. Similarly, supination is primarily inversion, but also includes some plantarflexion and forefoot adduction. These movements represent a 'twisting' of the forefoot (distal segment), relative to the hindfoot (proximal segment). However, some authorities regard pronation and supination as the basic movements and eversion and inversion as the combined movements. Increasingly the foot is being modelled in multiple segments, most commonly into three or four segments although more have been used. This requires further referencing of the relative movement of the different segments, which will be dealt with later in the chapter.

Bones

It could be argued that almost every bone in the body takes part in walking. However, from a practical point of view, it is generally only necessary to consider the bones of the pelvis and legs. These are shown in Figure 1.4.

The *pelvis* is formed from the sacrum, the coccyx and the two innominate bones. The *sacrum* consists of the five sacral vertebrae, fused together. The *coccyx* is the vestigial 'tail', made of three to five rudimentary vertebrae. The innominate bone on each side is formed by the fusion of three bones: the *ilium*, *ischium* and *pubis*. The only real movement between the bones of the pelvis occurs at the sacroiliac joint and this movement is generally very small in adults. It is thus reasonable, for the purposes of gait analysis, to regard the pelvis as being a single rigid structure.

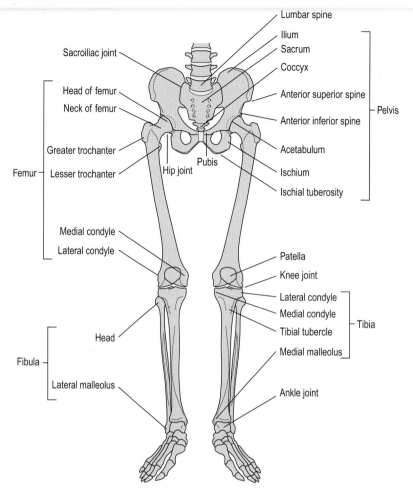

Fig. 1.4 • Bones and joints of the lower limbs.

The superior surface of the sacrum articulates with the fifth lumbar vertebra of the spine. On each side of the lower part of the pelvis is the acetabulum, which is the proximal part of the hip joint, being the socket into which the head of the femur fits.

The *femur* is the longest bone in the body. The spherical femoral head articulates with the pelvic acetabulum to form the hip joint. The neck of the femur runs downwards and laterally from the femoral head to meet the shaft of the bone, which continues downwards to the knee joint. At the junction of the neck and the shaft are two bony protuberances, where a number of muscles are inserted – the greater trochanter laterally, which can be felt beneath the skin, and the lesser trochanter medially. The bone widens at its lower end to form the medial and lateral condyles. These form the proximal part of the knee

joint and have a groove between them anteriorly, which articulates with the patella.

The *patella* or kneecap is a sesamoid bone; that is to say, it is embedded within a tendon, in this case the massive quadriceps tendon, which below the patella is known as the patellar tendon. The anterior surface of the patella is subcutaneous (immediately below the skin); its posterior surface articulates with the anterior surface of the lower end of the femur to form the patellofemoral joint. The patella has an important mechanical function, which is to displace the quadriceps tendon forwards, thereby improving its leverage.

The *tibia* extends from the knee joint to the ankle joint. Its upper end is broadened into medial and lateral condyles, with an almost flat upper surface which articulates with the femur. The tibial tubercle is a small bony prominence on the front of the tibia, where the patellar tendon is inserted. The anterior surface of the tibia is subcutaneous. The lower end of the tibia forms the upper and medial surfaces of the ankle joint, with a subcutaneous medial projection called the medial malleolus.

The *fibula* is next to the tibia on its lateral side. For most of its length it is a fairly slim bone, although it is broadened at both ends, the upper end being known as the head. The broadened lower end forms the lateral part of the ankle joint, with a subcutaneous lateral projection known as the lateral malleolus. The tibia and fibula are in contact with each other at their upper and lower ends, as the tibiofibular joints. Movements at these joints are very small and will not be considered further. A layer of fibrous tissue, known as the interosseous membrane, lies between the bones.

The foot is a very complicated structure (Fig. 1.5), which is best thought of as having four parts:

1. The *hindfoot*, which consists of two bones, one on top of the other
2. The *midfoot*, which consists of five bones, packed closely together
3. The *forefoot*, which consists of the five metatarsals
4. The toes, which consist of the five sets of phalangeal bones.

The *talus* or astragalus is the upper of the two bones in the hindfoot. Its superior surface forms the ankle joint, articulating above and medially with the tibia and laterally with the fibula. Below, the talus articulates with the calcaneus through the subtalar joint. It articulates anteriorly with the most medial and superior of the midfoot bones – the navicular.

The *calcaneus* or os calcis lies below the talus and articulates with it through the subtalar joint. Its lower surface transmits the body weight to the ground through a thick layer of fat, fibrous tissue and skin – the heelpad. The anterior surface articulates with the most lateral and inferior of the midfoot bones – the cuboid.

The midfoot consists of five bones:

1. The *navicular*, which is medial and superior
2. The *cuboid*, which is lateral and inferior
3. Three *cuneiform* bones (medial, intermediate and lateral), which lie in a row, distal to the navicular.

The five *metatarsals* lie roughly parallel to each other, the lateral two articulating with the cuboid and the medial three articulating with the three cuneiform bones.

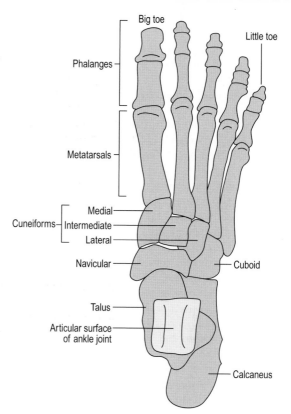

Fig. 1.5 • Bones of the right foot, seen from above.

The *phalanges* are the bones of the toes; there are two in the big toe and three in each of the other toes. The big toe is also called the great toe or hallux.

Joints and ligaments

A joint is the region where two bones come in contact with each other. From a practical point of view, they can be divided into synovial joints, in which significant movement can take place, and the various other types of joint in which only small movements can occur. Since gait analysis is usually only concerned with fairly large movements, the description which follows deals only with synovial joints. In a *synovial joint*, the bone ends are covered in *cartilage* and the joint is surrounded by a *synovial capsule*, which secretes the lubricant *synovial fluid*. Most joints are stabilised by *ligaments*, which are bands of relatively inelastic fibrous tissue connecting one bone to another. Fascia is a special type of connective tissue, being a continuous web of tissue found throughout the human body.

The *hip* joint is the only true ball-and-socket joint in the body, the ball being the head of the femur and the socket the acetabulum of the pelvis. Extremes of movement are prevented by a number of ligaments running between the pelvis and the femur, by a capsule surrounding the joint and by a small ligament – the ligamentum teres – which joins the centre of the head of the femur to the centre of the acetabulum. The joint is capable of flexion, extension, abduction, adduction, and internal and external rotation (Fig. 1.2).

The *knee* joint consists of the medial and lateral condyles of the femur, above, and the corresponding condyles of the tibia, below. The articular surfaces on the medial and lateral sides are separate, making the knee joint, in effect, two joints, side by side. The femoral condyles are curved both from front to back and from side to side, whereas the tibial condyles are almost flat. The 'gap' this would leave around the point of contact is filled, on each side, by a 'meniscus', commonly called a 'cartilage', which acts to spread the load and reduce the pressure at the point of contact.

The motion of the joint is controlled by five structures which, between them, exert very close control over the movements of the knee:

1. The medial collateral ligament (MCL), which prevents the medial side of the joint from opening up (i.e. it opposes abduction or valgus)
2. The lateral collateral ligament (LCL) similarly opposes adduction or varus
3. The posterior joint capsule, which prevents hyperextension (excessive extension) of the joint
4. The anterior cruciate ligament (ACL), in the centre of the joint, between the condyles; it is attached to the tibia anteriorly and the femur posteriorly. It prevents the tibia from moving forwards relative to the femur and also helps to prevent hyperextension of the knee as well as excessive internal rotation of the tibia
5. The posterior cruciate ligament (PCL), also in the centre of the joint, is attached to the tibia posteriorly and the femur anteriorly and prevents the tibia from moving backwards relative to the femur and also helps to limit external rotation of the tibia.

The anterior and posterior cruciate ligaments are named for the positions in which they are attached to the tibia. They appear to act together as what engineers call a 'four-bar linkage', which imposes a combination of sliding and rolling on the joint and moves the contact point forwards as the joint extends and backwards as it flexes. This means that the axis about which the joint flexes and extends is not fixed, but changes with the angle of flexion or extension. Pollo et al. (2003) challenged this description, saying that it only occurs in the unloaded knee and that during walking, the tibia moves backwards relative to the femur as the knee flexes.

In the normal individual, the motions of the knee are flexion and extension, with a small amount of internal and external rotation. Significant amounts of abduction and adduction are only seen in damaged knees. As the knee comes to full extension, there is an external rotation of a few degrees: the so-called automatic rotation or 'screw-home' mechanism.

The *patellofemoral* joint lies between the posterior surface of the patella and the anterior surface of the femur. The articular surface consists of a shallow V-shaped ridge on the patella, which fits into a shallow groove between the medial and lateral condyles. The principal movement is the patella gliding up and down in this groove, during extension and flexion of the knee, respectively. This causes different areas of the patella to come into contact with different parts of the joint surfaces of the femur. There is also some medial-lateral movement of the patella.

The *ankle* or talocrural joint has three surfaces: upper, medial and lateral. The upper surface is the main articulation of the joint; it is cylindrical and formed by the tibia above and the talus below. The medial joint surface is between the talus and the inner aspect of the medial malleolus of the tibia. Correspondingly, the lateral joint surface is between the talus and the inner surface of the lateral malleolus of the fibula.

The major ligaments of the ankle joint are those between the tibia and the fibula, preventing these two bones from moving apart, and the collateral ligaments on both sides, between the two malleoli and both the talus and calcaneus, which keep the joint surfaces in contact. The ankle joint, being cylindrical, has only one significant type of motion – dorsiflexion and plantarflexion – corresponding to flexion and extension in other joints.

The *subtalar* or talocalcaneal joint lies between the talus above and the calcaneus below. It has three articular surfaces: two anterior and medial and one posterior and lateral. Large numbers of ligaments join the two bones to each other and to all the adjacent bones. The axis of the joint is oblique, running primarily forwards but also upwards and medially. From a functional point of view, the importance of the subtalar joint is that it permits eversion/inversion (abduction and adduction or a valgus/varus motion) of the hindfoot. When performing gait analysis, it is usually impossible to distinguish between movement at the ankle joint and that taking place at the subtalar joint and it is reasonable to refer to motion taking place at the 'ankle/subtalar complex'. This motion in normal individuals includes dorsiflexion/ plantarflexion, hindfoot abduction/adduction, and internal/external rotation about the long axis of the tibia.

The *mid tarsal* joints lie between each of the tarsal bones and its immediate neighbours, making for a very complicated structure. The movement of most of these joints is very small, as there are ligaments crossing the joints and the joint surfaces are not shaped for large movements. As a result, the mid tarsal joints may be considered together to provide a flexible linkage between the hindfoot and the forefoot, which permits a small amount of movement in all directions.

The *tarsometatarsal* joints, between the cuboid and the cuneiforms proximally and the five metatarsals distally, are capable of only small gliding movements, because of the relatively flat joint surfaces and the ligaments binding the metatarsals to each other and to the tarsal bones. There are also joint surfaces between adjacent metatarsals, except for the medial one.

The *metatarsophalangeal* and *interphalangeal* joints consist of a convex proximal surface fitting into a shallow concave distal surface. The metatarsophalangeal joints permit abduction and adduction as well as flexion and extension; the interphalangeal joints are restricted by their ligaments to flexion and extension, the range of flexion being greater than that of extension. In walking, the most important movement in this region is extension at the metatarsophalangeal joints.

No description of the anatomy of the foot is complete without a mention of the arches. The bones of the foot are bound together by ligamentous structures, reinforced by muscle tendons, to make a flexible structure which acts like two strong curved springs, side by side. These are the longitudinal arches of the foot and they cause the body weight to be transmitted to the ground primarily through the calcaneus posteriorly and the metatarsal heads anteriorly. The midfoot transmits relatively little weight directly to the ground because it is lifted up, particularly on the medial side. The posterior end of both arches is the calcaneus. The *medial arch* (Fig. 1.6) goes upwards through the talus and then forwards and gradually down again through

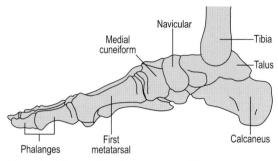

Fig. 1.6 • Medial side of the right foot. The medial arch consists of the calcaneus, talus, navicular, cuneiforms and medial three metatarsals.

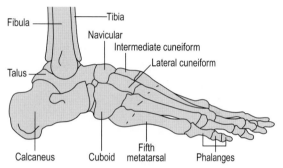

Fig. 1.7 • Lateral side of the right foot. The lateral arch consists of the calcaneus, cuboid and lateral two metatarsals.

the navicular and cuneiforms to the medial three metatarsals, which form the distal end of the arch. The *lateral arch* (Fig. 1.7) passes forwards from the calcaneus through the cuboid to the lateral two metatarsals.

Muscles and tendons

Muscles are responsible for movements at joints. Most muscles are attached to different bones at their two ends and cross over either one joint (*monarticular* muscle), two joints (*biarticular* muscle) or several joints (*polyarticular* muscle). In many cases the attachment to one of the bones covers a broad area, whereas at the other end it narrows into a *tendon*, which is attached to the other bone. It is usual to talk about a muscle as having an 'origin' and an 'insertion', although these terms are not always clearly defined. Ligaments and tendons are obviously similar and frequently confused. As a general rule, ligaments connect two bones together, whereas tendons connect muscles to bones.

The following is a brief account of the muscles of the pelvis and lower limb, including their major actions. Most muscles also have secondary actions, which may vary according to the position of the joints, particularly with biarticular muscles. The larger and more superficial muscles are illustrated in Figure 1.8.

Muscles acting only at the hip joint

1. *Psoas major* originates from the front of the lumbar vertebrae. Iliacus originates on the inside of the pelvis. The two tendons combine to form the iliopsoas, inserted at the lesser trochanter of the femur; the main action of these two muscles is to flex the hip.

2. *Gluteus maximus* originates from the back of the pelvis and is inserted into the back of the shaft of the femur near its top; it extends the hip.

3. *Gluteus medius* and *gluteus minimus* originate from the side of the pelvis and are inserted into the greater trochanter of the femur; they primarily abduct the hip.

4. *Adductor magnus*, *adductor brevis* and *adductor longus* all originate from the ischium and pubis of

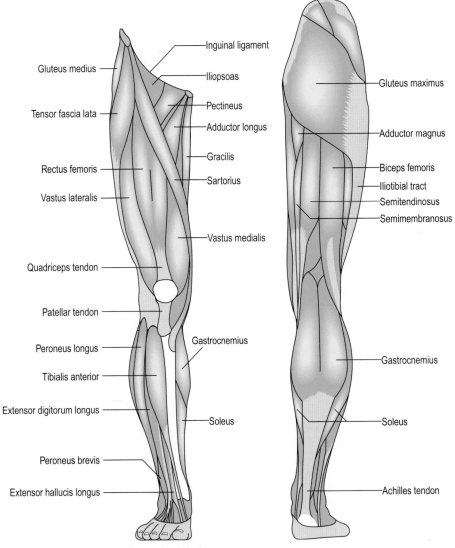

Fig. 1.8 • Superficial muscles of the right leg.

the pelvis. They insert in a line down the medial side of the femur and adduct the hip.

5. *Quadratus femoris, piriformis, obturator internus, obturator externus, gemellus superior* and *gemellus inferior* originate in the pelvis and insert close to the top of the femur; they all externally rotate the femur, although most also have secondary actions.

6. *Pectineus* originates on the pubis of the pelvis; it runs laterally and inserts on the front of the femur, near the lesser trochanter; it flexes and adducts the hip.

Internal rotation of the femur was not mentioned in the above list; it is achieved as a secondary action by gluteus medius, gluteus minimus, psoas major, iliacus, pectineus and tensor fascia lata (described below).

Muscles acting across the hip and knee joints

1. *Rectus femoris* originates from around the anterior inferior iliac spine of the pelvis and inserts into the *quadriceps* tendon; it flexes the hip, as well as being part of the quadriceps, a group of four muscles which extend the knee.

2. *Tensor fascia lata* originates from the pelvis close to the anterior superior iliac spine and is inserted into the iliotibial tract, a broad band of fibrous tissue which runs down the outside of the thigh and attaches to the head of the fibula. The muscle abducts the hip and the knee.

3. *Sartorius* is a strap-like muscle originating at the anterior superior iliac spine of the pelvis and winding around the front of the thigh, to insert on the front of the tibia on its medial side; it is mainly a hip flexor.

4. *Semimembranosus* and *semitendinosus* are two of the *hamstrings*; both originate at the ischial tuberosity of the pelvis and are inserted into the medial condyle of the tibia; they extend the hip and flex the knee.

5. *Biceps femoris* is the third hamstring; it has two origins – the 'long head' comes from the ischial tuberosity and the 'short head' from the middle of the shaft of the femur. It inserts into the lateral condyle of the tibia and is a hip extensor and knee flexor.

6. *Gracilis* runs down the medial side of the thigh from the pubis to the back of the tibia on its medial side; it adducts the hip and flexes the knee.

Muscles acting only at the knee joint

1. *Vastus medialis, vastus intermedius* and *vastus lateralis* are three elements of the quadriceps muscle. They all originate from the upper part of the femur, on the medial, anterior and lateral sides, respectively. The fourth element of the quadriceps is rectus femoris, described above. The four muscles combine to become the quadriceps tendon. This surrounds the patella and continues beyond it as the patellar tendon, which inserts into the tibial tubercle. Quadriceps is the only muscle which extends the knee.

2. *Popliteus* is a small muscle behind the knee; it flexes and helps to unlock the knee by internally rotating the tibia at the beginning of flexion.

Muscles acting across the knee and ankle joints

1. *Gastrocnemius* originates from the back of the medial and lateral condyles of the femur; its tendon joins with that of the soleus (and sometimes also the plantaris) to form the *Achilles tendon*, which inserts into the back of the calcaneus. The main action of these muscles is to plantarflex the ankle, although the gastrocnemius is also a flexor of the knee.

2. *Plantaris* is a very slender muscle running deep to the gastrocnemius from the lateral condyle of the femur to the calcaneus; it is a feeble plantarflexor of the ankle.

Muscles acting across the ankle and subtalar joints

1. *Soleus* arises from the posterior surface of the tibia, fibula and the deep calf muscles. Its tendon joins with that of the gastrocnemius (and sometimes plantaris) to plantarflex the ankle. The soleus and gastrocnemius together are called the *triceps surae*.

2. *Extensor hallucis longus, extensor digitorum longus, tibialis anterior* and *peroneus tertius* form the anterior tibial group. They originate from the anterior aspect of the tibia and fibula and the interosseous membrane. The former two are inserted into the toes, which they extend; the latter two are inserted into the tarsal bones and raise the midfoot on the medial side (tibialis anterior) or lateral side (peroneus tertius).

Tibialis anterior is the main ankle dorsiflexor; the others are weak dorsiflexors.

3. *Flexor hallucis longus, flexor digitorum longus, tibialis posterior, peroneus longus* and *peroneus brevis* are the deep calf muscles and all arise from the back of the tibia, fibula and interosseous membrane. The former two are flexors of the toes; the peronei are on the lateral side and evert the foot; tibialis posterior is on the medial side and inverts it. All five muscles are weak ankle plantarflexors.

Muscles within the foot

1. *Extensor digitorum* brevis and the *dorsal interossei* are on the dorsum of the foot; the former muscle extends the toes and the latter muscles abduct and flex the toes.
2. *Flexor digitorum brevis, abductor hallucis* and *abductor digiti minimi* form the superficial layer of the sole of the foot; they flex the toes and abduct the big toe and the little toe, respectively.
3. *Flexor accessorius, flexor hallucis brevis* and *flexor digiti minimi brevis* form an intermediate layer in the sole of the foot; between them they flex all the toes.
4. The *adductor hallucis* is in two parts – the oblique and transverse heads. It adducts the big toe.
5. The *plantar interossei* and the *lumbricals* lie in the deepest layer of the sole of the foot; the former adduct and flex the toes, the latter flex the proximal phalanges and extend the distal ones.

The above five groups of muscles are known together as the *intrinsic muscles* of the foot.

Spinal cord and spinal nerves

The *spinal cord* is an extension of the brain and plays an active role in the processing of nerve signals. Like the brain itself, it consists of white matter, which is bundles of nerve fibres, and grey matter, which contains many cell bodies and nerve endings, where the synapses (connections) between nerve cells take place. The spinal cord lies within the spinal canal, which is formed in front by the vertebral bodies and behind by the neural arches of the vertebrae (Fig. 1.9). The vertebrae are divided into four groups: cervical (7 vertebrae), thoracic (12), lumbar (5) and sacral (5). It is usual to use the abbreviated names, for example, the fourth thoracic vertebra is known as 'T4'.

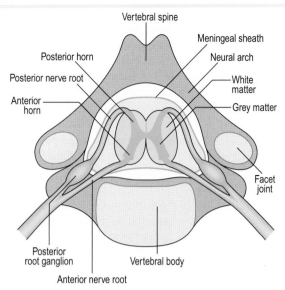

Fig. 1.9 • Cross-section of a vertebra, and the spinal cord and nerve roots.

The spinal cord is shorter than the spinal canal, terminating in adults at approximately the level of the first lumbar vertebra (L1) and in children a little lower. Beyond the end of the spinal cord is a bundle of nerves known as the *cauda equina*, which consists of the nerve roots that enter and leave the lower levels of the spinal canal (Fig. 1.10). There are eight cervical nerve roots but only seven cervical vertebrae; each nerve root except the eighth emerges above the correspondingly numbered vertebra. In the remainder of the spine, the nerve roots emerge below the correspondingly numbered vertebrae.

The organisation of the *neurons* (nerve cells) of the spinal cord and the peripheral nerves is extremely complicated. It is possible to give here only a brief outline, although further details will be given in the physiology section later in this chapter. The main neurons responsible for muscle contraction pass down from the brain as *upper motor neurons* in the 'descending' tracts of the spinal cord. At the appropriate spinal level, they enter the grey matter and connect with the *lower motor neurons*, also called *efferent* neurons. The axons (nerve fibres) of these cells pass out of the spinal cord through the *anterior root*, combine with other spinal roots and then split into smaller and smaller nerves, finally reaching the muscle itself.

Nerve fibres also pass in the opposite direction, from the muscles, skin and other structures to the spinal cord. They enter the spinal cord at the

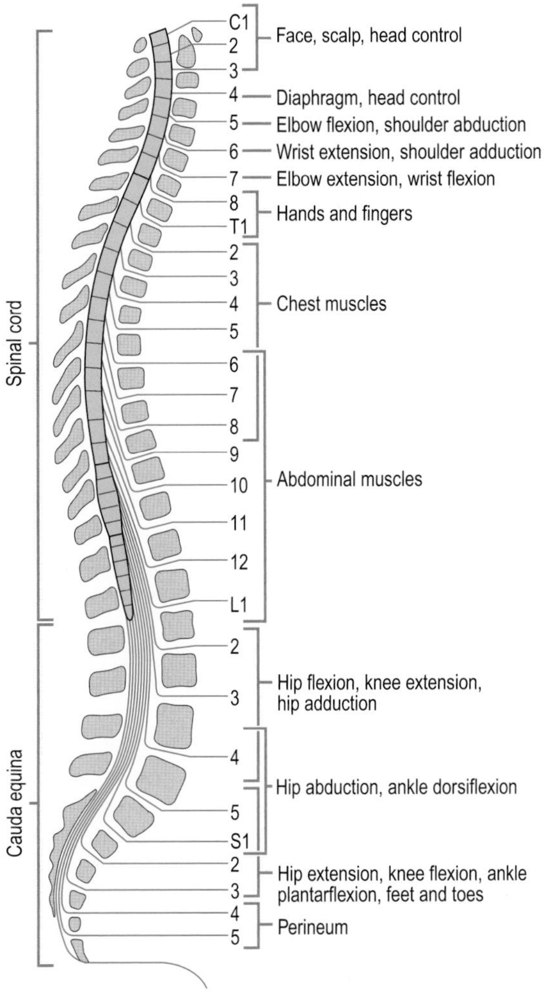
C1
2
3
Face, scalp, head control
4
Diaphragm, head control
5
Elbow flexion, shoulder abduction
6
Wrist extension, shoulder adduction
7
Elbow extension, wrist flexion
8
T1
Hands and fingers
2
3
4
5
Chest muscles
6
7
8
9
10
11
12
L1
Abdominal muscles
2
3
Hip flexion, knee extension, hip adduction
4
5
S1
Hip abduction, ankle dorsiflexion
2
3
Hip extension, knee flexion, ankle plantarflexion, feet and toes
4
5
Perineum
Spinal cord
Cauda equina

Fig. 1.10 • Spinal cord and spinal nerves, with main functions served.

posterior root, having passed through the *posterior root ganglion*, a swelling which contains the cell bodies of the neurons. These *afferent* neurons transmit many different types of sensory information. Some connect with the nerve fibres which pass up the spinal cord to the brain in the 'ascending' tracts, while others synapse with other nerve cells at the same or nearby spinal levels. Connections within the spinal cord are responsible for the spinal reflexes, which will be referred to later.

When the spinal cord is damaged by accident or disease, the results depend both on the spinal level at which the damage occurred and on whether the cord was totally or partially transected (cut through). A wide variety of disabilities may result from incomplete destruction of the spinal cord. If the cord is totally transected, the upper motor neurons are unable to control the muscle groups at or below that level, so voluntary control of those muscles is lost. There is also a total loss of sensation below the level of the damage. However, at levels below the damaged area, there is usually preservation of the lower motor neurons, the sensory nerves and the spinal reflexes. Injury to the vertebral column below L1 will damage the cauda equina, rather than the spinal cord. The cauda equina consists of lower motor neurons and sensory fibres and damage to it produces a totally different clinical picture from damage to the spinal cord itself.

Patients paralysed at the level of the cervical spine are *tetraplegic* or *quadriplegic*, with paralysis of the arms and legs. With a cervical lesion above C4, the diaphragm is also paralysed, making breathing difficult or impossible, and the chances of survival are poor. At the lower cervical levels, some arm or hand function is preserved. Where the spinal cord damage is at thoracic or lumbar level, only the legs are paralysed and the patient is *paraplegic*. Where only the cauda equina is damaged, the patient has an incomplete paraplegia and may be able to walk wearing some form of orthosis (an external support, also known as a brace or caliper). The word 'orthotic' was once synonymous with 'orthosis' but current usage restricts it to orthotic insoles, used within the shoes. Patients with paralysis restricted to one side of the body are *hemiplegic*. Sometimes the suffix '-paretic' may be used in place of '-plegic'; it implies an incomplete paralysis.

The area of skin served by the sensory nerves from a particular spinal root is known as a *dermatome*. The distribution of the dermatomes for all the spinal nerves is shown in Figure 1.11. In the legs, the anterior surface is innervated by the higher spinal segments and the posterior surface by the lower ones; loss of sensation from the buttocks and perineum is likely to follow spinal injury at almost any level.

Peripheral nerves

On emerging from the spinal cord, the spinal roots from adjacent levels form a network known as a *plexus*. The peripheral nerves which emerge from such a plexus usually contain nerve fibres from several adjacent spinal roots. The peripheral nerves supplying the muscles of walking all arise from either the

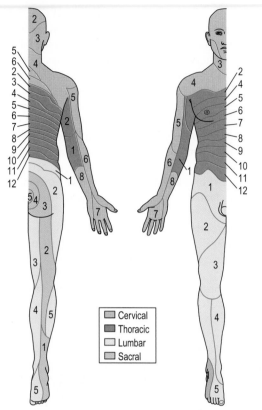

Cervical
Thoracic
Lumbar
Sacral

Fig. 1.11 • Sensory distribution (dermatomes) of the spinal nerve roots.

lumbar plexus or the *sacral plexus*. Table 1.1 gives brief details of the motor and sensory distribution of the nerves arising from the lumbar plexus and Table 1.2 the corresponding information for the nerves arising from the sacral plexus (sometimes called the lumbosacral plexus).

Physiology

Again, the following text is only intended to give an overview of the most important aspects of physiology which apply to gait. There are many good textbooks on the subject; the authors use Guyton (2005).

Nerves

Mention has already been made of the nerve cell or *neuron*, the basic element of the nervous system. Although neurons in different parts of the nervous system vary considerably in structure, they all consist of four basic elements (Fig. 1.12): *dendrites, cell body, axon* and *presynaptic endings*. Nerve impulses are conducted from the dendrites to the cell body and thence down the axon to the presynaptic endings. These contain very small packages of a chemical known as a *neurotransmitter*, which is released and crosses a small space known as a *synapse*, to stimulate the dendrite of another neuron. Within the brain and spinal cord, dendrites are stimulated to produce nerve impulses by the axons of other cells and in turn the nerve impulse sent along the axon stimulates the dendrites of other neurons. The peripheral nerves contain *motor neurons*, whose axons stimulate muscle fibres, and *sensory neurons*, in which the dendrites are stimulated by the sense organs.

The brain and spinal cord consist of millions of neurons, connected together in a vast and complex network. A single peripheral nerve consists of the axons and dendrites of hundreds or even thousands of individual neurons. The tissues of the brain, spinal cord and peripheral nerves also contain a number of other types of cell known as *neuroglia*, whose functions are either to provide physical support for the neurons or to perform a variety of maintenance functions.

The *upper motor neurons* arise in several different areas of the brain, but most notably in an area known as the motor cortex, and pass down the spinal cord to the appropriate level, crossing over to the other side at some point in their journey. Within the anterior horn of grey matter, the upper motor neurons synapse with the *lower motor neurons*, as well as with a large number of other neurons, which take part in the complex system of motor control.

The motor or efferent neurons arise in the anterior horns of the spinal cord, emerge from the anterior spinal roots and pass down the peripheral nerves to the muscles. The axon usually branches at its distal end, where it synapses with the muscle cells at a number of *motor endplates*. The nerve impulse causes contraction of the muscle, by a process which will be described later.

The *sensory nerves* arise in the sense organs of the skin, joints, muscles and other structures. The sense organ itself stimulates the end of the dendrite of the afferent neuron. The dendrite usually commences as a number of branches; these come together and run up the peripheral nerve to enter the posterior root of the spinal cord. The cell body is in the *posterior root ganglion* (Fig. 1.9) and the axon runs from this ganglion into the spinal cord itself, usually terminating in the posterior horn of grey matter, where it synapses with other neurons. As well as the familiar

Table 1.1 Distribution of nerves arising from the lumbar plexus

Nerve	Origin	Motor	Sensory
Anterior lumbar nerves	L2–3	Psoas major	
Iliohypogastric	T12–L1	Abdominal wall	Abdominal wall Lateral buttocks
Ilioinguinal	T12–L1	Abdominal wall	Abdominal wall Upper thigh Genitalia
Genitofemoral	L1–2	Genitalia	Upper thigh (anterior) Genitalia
Lateral femoral cutaneous	L2–3	–	Upper thigh (lateral)
Femoral	L2–4	Iliacus Pectineus Sartorius Rectus femoris Vastus lateralis Vastus intermedius Vastus medialis	Anterior thigh Medial thigh Medial leg Medial foot Hip joint Knee joint
Saphenous (branch of femoral nerve)	L2–4	–	Medial leg Medial foot Knee joint
Obturator	L2–4	Obturator externus Pectineus Adductor longus Adductor brevis Adductor magnus Gracilis	Medial thigh Hip joint Knee joint

sensations of touch, temperature, pain and vibration, sensory nerves also carry *proprioception* signals, which are used for feedback in the control of the limbs. These signals include the positions of the joints and the tension in the muscles and ligaments.

The term *nerve impulse* has been used above without explanation and it is now time to rectify this deficiency. The nature of the nerve impulse is a little difficult to grasp, since it is a complicated electrochemical process.

There are different concentrations of ions between the inside of cells (of all types) and the surrounding extracellular fluid. (Ions are atoms or molecules that have gained or lost one or more electrons, making them electrically charged.) The outside layer of a cell is known as the *cell membrane*; it is largely impermeable to sodium ions and any ions that leak in are 'pumped' out again. The inside of the cell contains large negatively charged ions, such as proteins, which are unable to pass through the cell membrane. The high concentration of positively charged sodium ions outside the cell, and of negative ions inside it, causes an automatic compensation, which results in a high concentration of potassium ions on the inside of the cell and of chloride ions outside. The inside of the cell thus has higher concentrations of potassium and large negative ions, while the outside has more sodium and chloride. The result of these imbalances in ionic concentration is a voltage difference between the inside and outside of the cell, across the thickness of the cell membrane. This membrane potential can be measured if a suitably small electrode is inserted. The normal resting *membrane potential* for a neuron is around -70 mV, the

13

Table 1.2 Distribution of nerves arising from the sacral plexus

Nerve	Origin	Motor	Sensory
Superior gluteal	L4–S1	Gluteus medius Tensor fascia lata	–
Inferior gluteal	L5–S2	Gluteus maximus	–
Nerve to piriformis	S1–2	Piriformis	–
Nerve to quadratus femoris	L4–S1	Quadratus femoris Inferior gemellus	Hip joint
Nerve to obturator internus	L5–S2	Obturator internus Superior gemellus	–
Perforating cutaneous	S2–3	–	Medial buttock
Posterior cutaneous	S1–3	–	Inferior buttock Posterior thigh Upper calf
Sciatic	L4–S3	Biceps femoris Semimembranosus Semitendinosus Adductor magnus	Knee joint
Tibial (branch of sciatic nerve)	L4–S3	Gastrocnemius Plantaris Soleus Popliteus Tibialis posterior Flex dig longus Flex hall longus	Lower leg (posterior) Posterior foot Lateral foot Knee joint Ankle joint
Medial plantar (branch of tibial nerve)		Abductor hallucis Flex dig brevis Flex hall brevis	Medial foot Distal toes Tarsal joints
Lateral plantar (branch of tibial nerve)		Remaining muscles of foot	Lateral foot Tarsal joints
Common peroneal (branch of sciatic nerve)	L4–S2	–	Knee joint
Superficial peroneal (branch of common peroneal nerve)		Peroneus longus Peroneus brevis	Anterior leg Dorsal foot
Deep peroneal (branch of common peroneal nerve)		Tibialis anterior Ext hall longus Ext dig brevis Ext dig longus Peroneus tertius	Great toe Second toe Ankle joint Tarsal joints
Pudendal	S2–4	Perineum	Genitalia

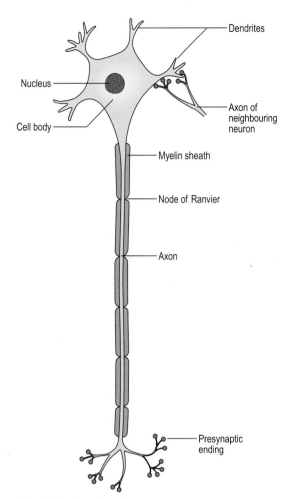

Fig. 1.12 • Structure of a neuron.

Labels (figure):
- Dendrites
- Nucleus
- Cell body
- Axon of neighbouring neuron
- Myelin sheath
- Node of Ranvier
- Axon
- Presynaptic ending

balance and returning the membrane potential to $-70\,mV$. The actual number of ions crossing the cell membrane is small and the overall composition of the cell is not affected to any appreciable extent; it is only when the sodium ions have entered, but before the potassium ions have left, that the membrane potential is reversed. This change in membrane potential by around $110\,mV$, from $-70\,mV$ to $+40\,mV$, is known as an *action potential*.

Under normal circumstances, an action potential in a neuron begins in the synapses, in response to the neurotransmitters released from the presynaptic endings of the axons of other neurons. Some of these are excitatory, which means that they reduce the membrane potential, and some are inhibitory, in that they increase it. This combination of excitatory and inhibitory influences permits the addition and subtraction of nerve impulses. If the net effect of the various excitatory and inhibitory influences causes the membrane potential to fall by around $20\,mV$, an action potential will occur in that region of the neuron. This action potential spreads from its origin, crossing the cell body and running down the axon to its termination.

The action potential is an 'all-or-none' phenomenon, its size and shape being independent of the intensity of the stimulus, provided it is above the threshold; there are no 'larger' or 'smaller' action potentials. However, the spacing of the action potentials may vary; a nerve can pass action potentials one after another, in quick succession, or only occasionally and separated by long intervals. Thus it is the frequency of the nerve impulses, not their size, which carries the information on how hard the muscle is to be contracted, for example, or on the temperature of the skin.

Figure 1.13 shows an action potential passing along an axon from left to right. At its leading edge, sodium ions enter the axon, producing a region with reversed polarity. At the trailing edge of the action potential, potassium ions leave the axon and the membrane potential is restored. The depolarised region has a membrane potential of $+40\,mV$, whereas the surrounding regions have a membrane potential of around $-70\,mV$. This is equivalent to a tiny battery producing $110\,mV$ and an electric current flows between the depolarised region and the surrounding normal regions of cell membrane. The passage of this electric current causes a drop in the membrane potential sufficient to generate an action potential in the normally polarised region in front, enabling the action potential to spread along the nerve. The region

negative sign indicating that the inside of the cell is negative with respect to the outside.

All body cells exhibit a membrane potential but nerve and muscle cells differ from other cells in that they can manipulate it, by altering the permeability of the cell membrane to sodium and potassium ions. This is the mechanism by which both nerve impulses and muscular contraction are propagated. If the membrane potential is lowered by about $20\,mV$, the membrane suddenly becomes extremely permeable to sodium ions, which enter rapidly from the extracellular fluid. While these ions are entering, the membrane potential is reversed to about $+40\,mV$ and it is said to be *depolarised*. The increase in permeability to sodium ions is short-lived and is followed by an increased permeability to potassium ions, which leave the cell, thus restoring the ionic

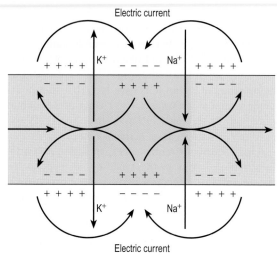

Electric current

Fig. 1.13 • Propagation of an action potential along an axon. Electric current flows from positive regions (+) to negative regions (–). The depolarised region is coloured green.

immediately behind an action potential becomes *refractory*, meaning that it cannot be stimulated again for a few milliseconds, so the action potential only moves in one direction.

The description so far has ignored the fact that many nerve fibres, particularly those required to send impulses quickly over long distances, are enclosed in a *myelin sheath*, as shown in Figure 1.12. Myelin is a fatty substance which surrounds nerve fibres, both axons and dendrites, as a series of sleeves, with gaps between them known as *nodes of Ranvier*. Since myelin is an insulator, it prevents the electric current from passing through the cell membrane close to an area of depolarisation, forcing it instead to pass through the next node of Ranvier, some distance along the nerve fibre. The effect of this is to cause the action potential to pass down the fibre in a series of jumps, known as *saltatory conduction*, which is much faster than the continuous propagation seen in unmyelinated fibres. A number of neurological diseases, most notably multiple sclerosis, are associated with loss of myelin from nerve fibres, with serious consequences to the functioning of the nervous system.

The speed at which nerve impulses travel depends on two things: the diameter of the nerve fibre and whether or not it is myelinated. Several types of fibres are found within the nervous system, known as types A, B and C. Type A fibres are all myelinated

and are further divided by their conduction velocities into three groups:

- A-alpha (α), 80–120 m/s
- A-beta (β), 35–75 m/s
- A-gamma (γ), 15–40 m/s
- A-delta (δ), 5–35 m/s.

Type B and C fibres are unmyelinated with conduction velocities around 10 m/s and 2 m/s, respectively. The type A fibres are the most important in gait analysis, especially the A-alpha fibres, which supply the motor nerves to muscles, and the A-beta and A-delta fibres, which conduct afferent impulses such as touch and/or pain. The gamma fibre is of particular importance in muscle physiology and will be referred to again later.

When an unmyelinated nerve fibre becomes damaged, recovery of function is usually impossible, because of the formation of scar tissue. For this reason, very little recovery of neuronal function takes place following damage to the brain or spinal cord, although function may be partially restored by the use of alternative neurological pathways. Myelinated fibres can recover, provided the cell body remains alive and the myelin sheaths remain in line; the nerve fibre regrows down the sheath at the rate of a few millimetres a week. In practice, if a complete nerve is divided and reconnected, most of the nerve fibres will enter the wrong myelin sheaths, although a sufficient number may be correctly connected to provide useful sensory and motor function.

Muscles

The human body contains three types of muscle: smooth, cardiac and skeletal. The description which follows is of *skeletal muscle*, also known as voluntary or striated muscle, which is responsible for the movement of the limbs.

A muscle is made up of hundreds of *fascicles* (Fig. 1.14), which in turn consist of hundreds of *muscle fibres*. These large multinucleated cells (cells with many nuclei) are the basic units of muscle tissue. The fibre is itself made up of hundreds of *myofibrils*, which have a characteristic striated (striped) appearance. The striations are due to a regular arrangement of *filaments*, which are made of two types of protein – *actin* and *myosin*. It is the sliding of these filaments past each other, by the formation and destruction of cross-bridges, which is responsible for muscle contraction.

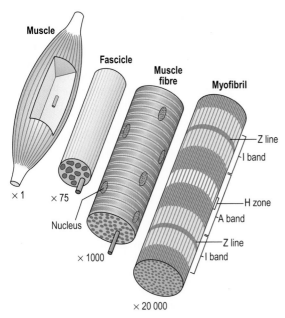

Fig. 1.14 • Macroscopic and microscopic structure of muscle.

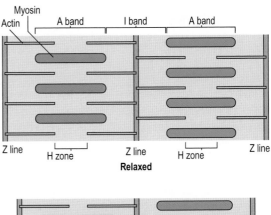

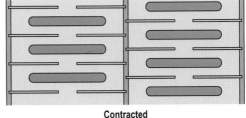

Fig. 1.15 • Sliding of actin and myosin filaments during muscular contraction.

The various light and dark bands in the myofibril are identified by letters. The thin, dark 'Z' line is the origin of the slender actin filaments (Fig. 1.15). These are interleaved with the thicker myosin filaments, which form the 'A' band. The 'I' band and 'H' zone change their width during muscular contraction, as they represent the areas where the actin and myosin, respectively, are *not* overlapped – they were named before the process of contraction was understood!

There is an extremely complicated arrangement of membranes surrounding the myofibrils within the muscle fibre. It is responsible for the transport of nutrients and waste products and the transmission of the muscle action potential. Outside the muscle fibres are the blood capillaries and the terminal branches of the motor nerves, which connect to the muscle fibres at *motor endplates*, also known as neuromuscular junctions. On average, a single motor nerve will connect to about 150 muscle fibres, the combination of the neuron and the muscle fibres it innervates being known as a *motor unit*.

When an action potential passes down a nerve to the motor endplate, it results in the release of the transmitter substance *acetylcholine* (ACH). ACH diffuses across the synaptic cleft and binds to receptors on the muscle cell membrane causing depolarisation of the membrane, which causes a spreading wave of depolarisation. As this *muscle action potential* spreads throughout the muscle fibre, it causes the release of calcium ions, which trigger muscle contraction. Cross-bridges form between the actin and myosin molecules, pulling them together. The tension is maintained for a brief period, then released if no further action potential occurs, the calcium ions being removed by the *calcium pump*. The electrical activity of muscle action potentials can be detected and is known as the *electromyogram* (EMG).

The energy for muscular contraction comes from the release of a high-energy phosphate group from a chemical known as *adenosine triphosphate* (ATP). The regeneration of ATP requires the expenditure of metabolic energy and a failure to keep up with the demand results in muscle fatigue. There are two metabolic pathways involved in regeneration of ATP. One uses up chemicals stored within the cell (phosphocreatine and glucose), without the need for oxygen, and is known as *anaerobic*; the other requires oxygen and nutrients to enter the muscle fibre from the bloodstream and is known as *aerobic*. Anaerobic processes are quickly exhausted, although they can provide brief bursts of powerful contraction. For more sustained muscular effort, aerobic metabolism is required. Following anaerobic respiration, a muscle will have an *oxygen debt*, which will need to

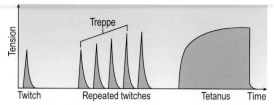

Fig. 1.16 • Response of a single muscle fibre to single stimulation and to repeated stimulation at low and high frequencies.

be 'repaid' by aerobic respiration, to remove lactic acid, which accumulates in the muscle.

If a single nerve impulse stimulates a muscle, it will respond, after a short pause known as the *latent period*, with a brief contraction known as a *twitch* (Fig. 1.16). If the motor nerve delivers a second nerve impulse during the latent period, it has no effect. The force which a muscle is able to generate in a contraction depends on a number of factors, particularly the strength of stimulation, the cross-sectional area of the muscle, the speed of contraction and the direction of contraction. The greatest force is usually produced when the muscle length is close to its middle range of length. If a muscle shortens to its minimum length, its force of contraction falls greatly ('*active insufficiency*'). If the muscle becomes stretched over two or more joints it may be unable to stretch enough to complete full range of motion in both joints simultaneously. This is termed 'passive insufficiency'. An example of this is that when the wrist is fully flexed with the fingers extended it becomes impossible to then fully flex the fingers as the finger extensor tendons have been stretched over several joints and cannot elongate further.

There are a number of different types of muscle fibre, the main subdivision being into types I and II. The type of muscle fibre depends on the nerve innervating it. Because of this, all the fibres in a single motor unit are of the same type. *Type I fibres* (slow twitch) are dark in colour, they contract and relax slowly and are fatigue resistant; they are used primarily for the sustained contractions used for posture control. *Type II fibres* (fast twitch) are pale in colour, quick to contract and relax, and easily fatigued. They are mainly used for brief bursts of powerful contraction. Depending on their function in the body, different muscles have different proportions of fast and slow fibres. This is also seen in poultry, where the 'red meat' in the leg muscles is used for sustained contraction and the 'white meat' in the wing muscles is used for bursts of powerful contraction. A change in the stimulation pattern will cause a change in the fibre type in the course of a few weeks, despite the fact that the fibre types differ in the actual structure of the myosin. This ability to alter the fibre type becomes very important when electrical stimulation is used on paralysed muscles.

When a muscle contracts, not all the motor units are active at the same time. If a stronger contraction is needed, further motor units are brought into use, a process known as *recruitment*.

If a muscle generates tension without changing its length, the contraction is known as *isometric*. If the muscle changes its length but the force of contraction remains the same, the contraction is *isotonic*. One normally thinks of a muscle shortening as it contracts – a *concentric contraction*. However, it is quite usual, particularly in gait, for a muscle to produce tension while it is lengthening – an *eccentric contraction*. For example, the quadriceps undergoes an eccentric contraction as you sit down. The muscle which is responsible for a particular action is known as an *agonist*. If two or more muscles act together, they are known as *synergists*; muscles which oppose agonists are known as *antagonists*. As a general rule, contraction of one set of muscles results in *reciprocal inhibition* of opposing muscles.

Muscle atrophy is the term used to describe the loss of bulk and strength of a muscle when it is not used. If the motor nerve is intact, the muscle fibres will become smaller but their numbers remain the same and subsequent restoration of muscle stimulation will lead to a full recovery of function. This happens, for example, when a limb is encased in plaster following a fracture. This type of muscle atrophy also occurs in spinal cord injury where the upper motor neurons are destroyed but the lower motor neurons remain intact. In contrast, if the lower motor neuron is destroyed, the muscle fibres shrink and become replaced by fibrous tissue. This leads to an irreversible form of muscle atrophy, such as is seen following poliomyelitis and after damage to the cauda equina or peripheral nerves.

Spinal reflexes

The lower motor neurons receive nerve impulses from both the brain and other neurons within the spinal cord. The two areas of the brain chiefly concerned with posture and movement are the *motor cortex*, which is responsible for voluntary movement, and the *cerebellum*, which is responsible for generating patterns of muscular activity. The motor cortex and its associated nerves are known as the *pyramidal system*; the cerebellum and some associated brain centres, with their associated nervous pathways, are known as the *extrapyramidal system*. Within the spinal cord itself, the influences of other neurons give rise to the *spinal reflexes*. There are also pattern generators for each limb within the spinal cord, which are capable of producing alternating flexion and extension.

The brain and higher centres exert an inhibitory influence on spinal reflexes, which as a result are often very weak in normal individuals. However, the reflexes may become very strong, due to the loss of this inhibition, in patients who have suffered damage to the brain or spinal cord.

One of the most important spinal reflexes (for the spinal nerve L4) is the *stretch reflex*, which is responsible for the knee-jerk, when the patellar tendon is struck by a small hammer. When a muscle is stretched, *stretch receptors* within it are stimulated, sending nerve impulses to the spinal cord along fast sensory neurons. Within the cord, these neurons synapse with and stimulate the lower motor neurons of the same muscle, causing it to contract. The stretch receptors are within the *muscle spindles* and attached to very small *intrafusal muscle fibres*, which are innervated by thin, relatively slow *gamma motor neurons*. These adjust the length of the spindle as the main muscle contracts and relaxes, so that it continues to work over the complete range of muscle lengths. The intrafusal fibres are also able to alter the 'sensitivity' of the stretch receptor. The stretch reflex provides a feedback system for maintaining the position of a muscle despite changes in the force applied to it. The stretch reflex is unusual in that it involves only a single synapse, between the sensory and motor neurons, making it a *monosynaptic reflex*. Most reflexes are *polysynaptic*, involving many intermediate neurons and often involving neurons on both sides of the spinal cord and at more than one spinal level.

Partly because of the stretch reflex and partly through a continuous low level of activity in the motor neurons, most muscles show a certain amount of resistance to being stretched – this is known as *muscle tone*. In some individuals this effect is exaggerated, giving the clinical condition of *spasticity*, in which muscle tone is very high, small movements of the limb being opposed by strong muscular contractions.

Spasticity is an important cause of gait abnormalities. It usually results from the loss of some or all of the inhibitory influence of the higher centres on the spinal reflexes and is often seen in patients with brain damage (as in cerebral palsy) or following damage to the spinal cord. A related phenomenon, also seen in gait, is *clonus* in which a muscle produces a series of contractions, one after the other, in response to being stretched.

Many different types of sensory organ in the tissues are responsible for spinal reflexes, those of particular importance in gait analysis being the muscle spindle, referred to above, and the *Golgi organ*. The latter is a stretch receptor in tendons which inhibits muscular contraction if the force applied to the tendon, either actively or passively, becomes dangerously large. Pain receptors in the limb may elicit the *flexor withdrawal reflex*, in which the flexor muscles contract and the extensors relax, hopefully to remove the limb from whatever is causing the pain. There is also a *crossed extensor reflex*, where contraction of flexors on one side is accompanied by contraction of extensors on the other. An example of this is a person who has stepped on a nail with their right foot; the right leg flexes to move away from the pain and the left leg extends to hold the full body weight up.

Motor control

Walking is accomplished through a complex and coordinated pattern of nerve signals, sent to the muscles, which in turn move the joints, the limbs and the remainder of the body. The 'central pattern generator', which produces this pattern of nerve impulses, is not located in a single place but consists of networks of neurons in various parts of the brain and spinal cord. Much of the research in this area has been done on experimental animals but there is some evidence that human locomotion is organised in a similar fashion to that in cats, where a rhythm-generating system within the spinal cord is controlled by neural input from 'higher levels' in the brain and receives feedback from sensors in the muscles, joints and skin of the legs (Duysens and Van de Crommert, 1998).

Biomechanics

Biomechanics is a scientific discipline which studies biological systems, such as the human body, by the methods of mechanical engineering. Since gait is a mechanical process which is performed by a biological system, it is appropriate to study it in this way. Mechanical engineering is a vast subject but the descriptions which follow are limited to those aspects which are most relevant to gait analysis, especially time, mass, force, centre of gravity, moments of force, and motion, both linear and angular. The science of biomechanics can be extremely mathematical, but the basic principles are easy to grasp and the section ends with a worked example to illustrate this. A good text on the scientific basis of movement is Richards (2008).

Time

The second (s) and the millisecond (ms) are the primary units for time measurement in biomechanics, although it is still fairly common to find walking speed quoted in metres per minute or even miles per hour. When repeated events occur at short intervals of time, it is usual to quote a 'frequency' in hertz (abbreviated 'Hz'), 1 Hz being one cycle per second. For example, a typical gait analysis system might measure the positions of markers on a patient's limbs at 100 Hz (corresponding to an interval between samples of 10 ms), the ground reaction force at 500 Hz (2 ms interval between samples) and EMG at 2000 Hz (0.5 ms interval between samples). The relationship between sample interval and frequency is given by:

$$\text{Interval (ms)} = 1000/\text{frequency (Hz)}$$

Mass

As we all live in the Earth's gravitational field, we normally use the terms mass and weight to mean the same thing. However, there is a clear distinction between them. The mass of an object is the amount of matter contained in it, which does not depend on whether any gravity is present, whereas weight is the force exerted by gravity on the object. For example, in an orbiting spacecraft there is no gravity and all objects are weightless, although they still have *mass*. This means that you are still likely to be injured if someone throws a moon-rock at you inside a spacecraft, even though it doesn't 'weigh' anything! We casually talk about measuring our body *'weight'* in kilograms (kg) or pounds but this is incorrect in scientific terms, as these are units of mass, not of force. As an example, a man with a mass of 90 kg (198 lb) has a weight of 882.9 N (90 kg * 9.81 m/s^2).

Force

We are all familiar in general terms with the concept of force but the scientist uses the term in a particular way. Force is a *vector* quantity, which means that it has both magnitude and direction, in contrast to *scalar* quantities, such as temperature, which have only magnitude. The internationally agreed system for scientific measurement is the Système International (SI). The unit of force in this system is the *newton* (N). The force applied by normal earth gravity to a mass of 1 kg is 9.81 N; 1 N is the force exerted by gravity on a mass of about 102 g or 3½ ounces. This is easily visualised as being the weight of an average size apple! The earlier imperial and metric units of force were confusing and are best avoided; for conversions, see Appendix 2). The direction of a force vector may be stated in any convenient manner, for example 20 N downwards or 140 N at 30° to the x-axis. However, the direction should never be omitted, unless it is obvious.

The whole science of mechanical engineering is based on the three laws of force propounded by Sir Isaac Newton, which may be paraphrased as follows.

Newton's first law

A body will continue in a state of rest, or of uniform motion in a straight line, unless it is acted upon by an external force.

Newton's second law

An external force will cause a body to accelerate in the direction of the force. The acceleration (*a*) is equal to the size of the force (*F*) divided by the mass (*m*) of the object, as in the equation:

$$F = m * a$$

Newton's third law

To every action there is a reaction, which is equal in magnitude and opposite in direction.

Neglecting the strange behaviour of atomic and subatomic particles, all physical systems simultaneously obey all three of Newton's laws.

It is easy to remember which law is which if you first imagine a brick, just floating in space (first law); then someone pushes it and it accelerates (second law); as it is accelerating, the brick pushes back on whoever or whatever is pushing it (third law).

It is easy to see that a single force acting in one direction can be balanced out by an equal force acting in the opposite direction. A much more common situation, however, is to have a number of forces acting in different directions which, taken together, balance out each other. Provided that direction is taken into account, it is possible to add and subtract force vectors, as it is with any other vectors such as velocity or acceleration. To understand how this is possible, it is necessary to appreciate the fact that a single force, acting in a single direction, can be exactly equivalent to a number of different forces acting in other directions. Conversely, any number of separate forces can be represented by an appropriate single force.

The technique used to convert a single force into two forces, acting in different directions, is known as *resolving into components*. Figure 1.17 shows how the resultant force F can be represented by two smaller forces, F_x and F_y, acting at right angles to each other. The magnitude of these forces is given by the formulae:

$$F_x = F \times \cos A$$
$$F_y = F \times \sin A$$

where A is the angle between the resultant force F and F_x.

The converse process (i.e. the combination of F_x and F_y to yield the resultant F), can be performed using these formulae:

$$\text{Magnitude: } F = \sqrt{\left(F_x{}^2 + F_y{}^2\right)}$$
$$\text{Angle A} = \tan^{-1}\left(F_y/F_x\right)$$

In order to combine forces, they are first resolved into components, using a common system of directions. Next, all the x components are added together and so are all the y components. The resulting totals are then used to find the single equivalent force. This is illustrated in Figure 1.18, where two forces, F_a and F_b represent resultant muscle forces acting around the hip joint. First, F_a and F_b are resolved into components ($F_{a\ x}$, $F_{a\ y}$, $F_{b\ x}$ and $F_{b\ y}$). The algebraic sum of the x components gives the x component of the resultant force acting on the hip joint and similarly with the y components. Since $F_{a\ x}$ and $F_{b\ x}$ are in opposite directions, their algebraic sum is actually their difference. The resultant, R, is then obtained by recombining the x and y components.

It follows from Newton's second law that if an object is not accelerating, there can be no net force acting on it. Any forces which are acting on the object must be balanced out by other, equal and opposite forces. If the forces do not appear to balance, yet the object is not accelerating or decelerating, there must be at least one force which has not been taken into account.

Figure 1.19A shows an individual standing perfectly still. In this case the ground reaction force will be equal and opposite to the weight of the person and will be acting only in a vertical direction with no horizontal component. However if we consider the forces during walking, in late stance phase there is a horizontal force F_x which is unopposed which will cause an acceleration or propulsion of the body forwards (Fig. 1.19B). We can also see that the vertical force F_y is greater than the weight of the person causing an acceleration of the body upwards.

Centre of gravity

Although the mass of any object is distributed throughout every part of it, it is frequently convenient, as far as the effects of an applied force are concerned, to imagine that the whole mass is concentrated at a single point. This point, which should be called the centre of mass is usually called

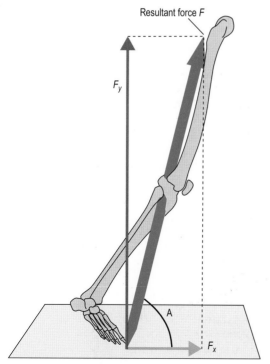

Fig. 1.17 • Resolution of force F into two components at right angles: F_x and F_y.

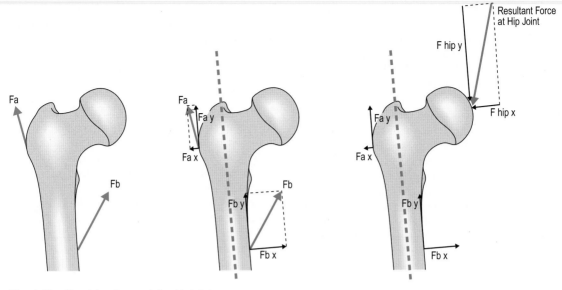

Fig. 1.18 • Resolving forces at the hip joint.

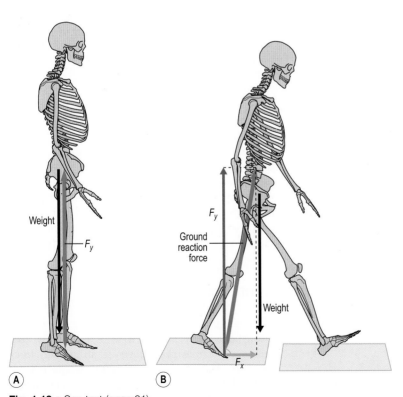

Fig. 1.19 • See text (page 21)

the *centre of gravity*. For a regular shape, such as a cube, made of a uniform material, it is easy to see that the centre of gravity must be at the geometric centre. However, for irregular and changing shapes, such as the human body, it may be necessary to determine it by direct measurement. It is also possible to determine the centre of gravity of every part of the body separately and to find the centre of gravity of the whole body by adding these together (by a method which is beyond the scope of this book). It is frequently stated that the centre of gravity of the body is just in front of the lumbosacral junction. This is approximately true for a person standing in the anatomical position but any movement of the body will move the centre of gravity. It is not even necessary for the centre of gravity to remain within the body; the centre of gravity of someone bending down to touch their toes will usually be outside the body, in front of the top of the thigh (Fig. 1.20). An interesting example of this is the technique used by skilled high-jumpers, who curve the body in such a way that although each part of the body in turn passes over the bar, the centre of gravity actually passes *under* it!

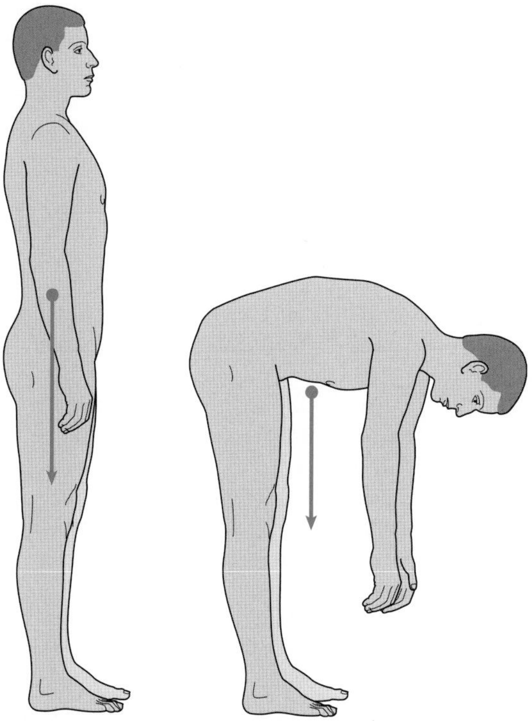

Moment of force

If an adult wishes to play with a small child on a seesaw, they will have to sit much closer to the pivot in order to balance the weight of the child (Fig. 1.21). The action which tends to unbalance the seesaw is the *moment of force*, which is calculated by multiplying the magnitude of the force by its perpendicular distance from the fulcrum or pivot point, this distance commonly being referred to as the *lever arm* or *moment arm*. The 'moment of force' may also be referred to as the 'torque', the 'turning moment' or simply the 'moment'. The formula for calculating the moment of force is:

$$M = F \times D$$

where M is the moment of force (in newton-metres, N·m), F is the force (in newtons, N) and D is the distance (in metres, m).

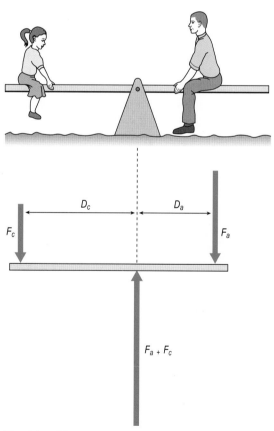

Fig. 1.20 • Centre of gravity when standing and when bending.

Fig. 1.21 • The adult on the seesaw will balance the child if the force F_a multiplied by the distance D_a equals the force F_c multiplied by the distance D_c.

For the system to be in equilibrium (that is, for the seesaw to balance), *the sum of the clockwise moments of force must equal the sum of the anticlockwise moments*. In Figure 1.21, if the child has a mass of 40 kg, she will exert a force due to gravity (F_c) of:

$$40 \text{ kg} \times 9.81 \text{ m/s}^2 = 392.4 \text{ N}$$

If her distance (D_c) from the fulcrum is 4 m, she exerts an anticlockwise moment of:

$$392.4 \text{ N} \times 4 \text{ m} = 1569.6 \text{ N·m}$$

A 70 kg adult will produce a downward force (F_a) of:

$$70 \text{ kg} \times 9.81 \text{ m/s}^2 = 686.7 \text{ N}$$

This will produce an opposing clockwise moment of 1569.6 N·m if he sits at a distance (D_a) from the fulcrum of:

$$1569.6 \text{ N·m}/686.7 \text{ N} = 2.29 \text{ m}$$

The definition of a moment of force refers to the perpendicular distance from the fulcrum. This is very important if opposing moments are produced by forces which act in different directions. Figure 1.22 illustrates the moments of force about the knee joint when standing with the knee bent. The ground reaction force is acting at a perpendicular distance 'a' from the point of loadbearing. The quadriceps tendon is pulling at an oblique angle relative to the vertical and the moment of force it provides is the product of the tension in the tendon and the perpendicular distance 'b'. It will be

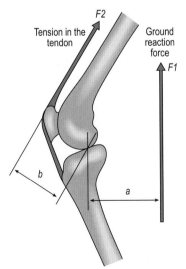

F2
Tension in the tendon
Ground reaction force
F1
b
a

Fig. 1.22 • The moment of force due to ground reaction force, F_1 multiplied by a, is opposed by contraction of the quadriceps, producing a moment of force F_2 multiplied by b.

noted that the presence of the patella increases the value of b and hence reduces the muscle force needed to produce a given moment of force. For equilibrium, the two moments ($F_1 \times a$) and ($F_2 \times b$) must be equal.

The measurement and interpretation of moments of force are essential for the full understanding of normal and pathological gait. 'Active' internal moments are generated by muscular contraction (concentric, isometric or eccentric). 'Passive' internal moments are generated by bone-on-bone forces and by tension in the soft tissues, especially ligaments. Moments may also be transmitted from adjacent joints. External moments (sometimes referred to as 'reaction moments') are generally due to gravitational forces. Modern gait analysis systems are able to measure the 'net moment' at the major joints during walking, which is the sum of all the active and passive moments present. However, this is seldom used to calculate the contraction force of a particular muscle, because there is frequently more than one muscle contracting. An example of this is 'co-contraction' at the hip joint, where flexor and extensor muscles contract at the same time, to increase the stability of the joint (Park et al., 1999).

Unfortunately, some confusion exists in the literature, because a term such as 'flexor moment' is often used without stipulating whether it refers to an internal or external moment. Contraction of a flexor muscle generates an *internal* flexor moment. In contrast, an *external* flexor moment attempts to flex the joint and is likely to be resisted by the contraction of extensor muscles (an example would be landing from a jump and the knee flexing from the force; the knee extensors would resist this external moment and prevent excessive knee flexion). To avoid such confusion, it is essential to make it clear whether any moment is internal or external. The gait analysis community now tends to use internal moments, a convention which has been adopted in this book, although the important textbook by Perry (1992) used external moments.

A *couple* is a moment that is produced by two equal forces which are parallel to each other but acting in opposite directions. The forces cancel each other out as far as producing linear motion is concerned (displacement or acceleration) but work together to produce rotation about a point between them.

In the same way that Newton's third law states that every force is opposed by another 'equal and opposite' force, every moment of force is opposed by an equal and opposite moment. It is impossible to generate a moment unless there is something to 'push back' with an opposing moment. The consequence of this for gait analysis is that if an external force generates a moment at a particular joint (attempting to flex the knee, for example), there *must* be a corresponding internal moment, generated within the joint, to oppose it. In the case of the knee, only the quadriceps muscles can provide an internal extensor moment, although for most joints both muscles and stretched ligaments can generate internal moments.

Any object which is supported by the ground will remain stable so long as the *line of gravity* (the line of force passing vertically downwards from the centre of gravity) remains within the area on the ground which is supporting it. Should the line of gravity stray outside this area, one of two things can happen: it may automatically correct itself, as happens with a self-righting lifeboat, or it may fall over, as will happen with a pencil balanced on its point. The former is a *stable equilibrium*, where a degree of imbalance produces 'restoring' moments, which push the object back towards the balanced position. The latter is an *unstable equilibrium*, where the moments act to increase the imbalance. When walking at moderate speeds, a further condition exists – a *dynamic equilibrium*, where from instant to instant the equilibrium is unstable but before there has been time to fall, the area of support is moved and equilibrium is restored.

The measurement of the moments generated about the joints of the lower limbs is an important part of scientific gait analysis. Such moments may be expressed in their original units (e.g. newton-metres) or they may be 'normalised' by dividing by body mass, changing the units to newton-metres per kilogram, to make it easier to compare results between individuals of different sizes. Although there is no general agreement on the best method of accomplishing such normalisation (Pierrynowski and Galea, 2001; Stansfield et al., 2003), it seems reasonable to normalise forces with reference to body mass and moments with reference to both body mass and either height or limb length.

Linear motion

The *velocity* of a moving object is the rate at which its position changes, which usually means the distance it covers in a given time. This is, of course, similar to the everyday concept of speed, except that velocity is a vector and thus has direction as well as magnitude. In measuring gait, the usual unit for velocity is metres per second, which can be abbreviated to either m/s or $m \cdot s^{-1}$. Sometimes other units are used, such as metres per minute or kilometres per hour, but the SI units are to be preferred.

Acceleration is the rate at which velocity changes; the change may be in either magnitude or direction. An unchanging velocity has an acceleration of zero; a decrease in velocity may be known as negative acceleration, deceleration or retardation. If the velocity is measured in metres per second, the acceleration will be in metres per second per second, abbreviated to m/s^2 or $m \cdot s^{-2}$. The acceleration due to gravity has already been mentioned; it has a value of 9.81 m/s^2.

The relationships between velocity, acceleration and distance travelled are given by four equations:

$$v = u + at$$
$$s = \frac{1}{2}(ut + vt)$$
$$s = ut + \frac{1}{2}at^2$$
$$v^2 - u^2 = 2as$$

where u is the initial velocity (in metres per second, m/s)

v is the final velocity (in metres per second, m/s)

a is the acceleration (in metres per second per second, m/s^2)

t is the time (in seconds, s)

s is the distance travelled (in metres, m).

These equations help us to find unknown distances, velocities and accelerations. However all these equations assume acceleration is constant and therefore care is needed when using them in human movement and in particular gait analysis where this is seldom the case.

Circular motion

An object which is rotating has an *angular velocity* and if the angular velocity changes, there is an *angular acceleration*, such as when a wheel, rotating on its axle, either speeds up or slows down. In walking, the leg has an angular velocity and undergoes angular acceleration and retardation. Every rotating object has an angular velocity, even if it is not attached to an axle or fulcrum, and a change in that angular velocity is an angular acceleration. In the same way that linear acceleration depends on the presence of a force, angular acceleration will only occur if there is an application of a moment of force.

The detailed mathematics of angular velocity and angular acceleration are beyond the scope of this book, but it is worth saying a few words about the general concepts. Angular velocity is measured by the angle turned per unit time, usually in degrees per second or radians per second. Angular acceleration is similarly expressed in degrees (or radians) per second per second. The radian is an obscure unit to non-mathematicians; it is the ratio, within the arc of a circle, of the length of the arc to the radius of the circle. There are 2π radians in a complete circle, giving the relationship:

$$1 \text{ rad} = 180°/\pi = 57.296°$$

When a force applied to an object produces an angular acceleration, the acceleration does not depend solely on the size of the force and the mass of the object, as it does with linear motion. It also depends on the way in which the mass is distributed about the centre of gravity, a property known as the *moment of inertia*. An object with the mass concentrated around the outside, such as a flywheel, has a much higher moment of inertia than one with the mass concentrated around the centre, such as a cannon ball. If a flywheel and a cannon ball have the same mass and are spinning with the same angular velocity, the flywheel will be much more difficult to stop rotating than the cannon ball, because of its higher moment of inertia.

Inertia and momentum

The term *inertia* is used to describe the resistance offered by a body to any attempt to set it in motion or to stop it if it is already moving. It is a descriptive term, rather than a measured physical quantity. In the case of linear motion, it results from the mass of the object; in the case of rotational motion, it results from the moment of inertia.

Momentum exists in two forms – linear and angular. The *linear momentum* (generally just called 'momentum') of a moving object is calculated by multiplying its velocity by its mass. A force applied to the object will cause it to change its velocity and hence its momentum. Another way of expressing Newton's second law is to say that the force is equal to the rate of change of momentum. The *angular momentum* of a rotating object is calculated by multiplying its angular velocity by its moment of inertia. A law of conservation of momentum exists, which states that momentum (both linear and angular) cannot be created or destroyed, merely transferred from one object to another.

Momentum has received little attention in gait analysis in the past but transfers of momentum are involved at a number of key events of the gait cycle, including the heelstrike transient and the end of the swing phase, both of which will be described in more detail in Chapter 2.

Kinetics and kinematics

The terms kinetics and kinematics are commonly used in gait analysis and they deserve some explanation. *Kinetics* is the study of forces, moments, masses and accelerations, but without any detailed knowledge of the position or orientation of the objects involved. For example, an instrument known as a force platform is used in gait analysis to measure the force beneath the foot during walking, but it gives no information on the position of the limb or the angle of the joints. *Kinematics* describes motion, but without reference to the forces involved. An example of a kinematic instrument is a video camera, which can be used to observe the motion of the trunk and the limbs during walking, but which gives no information on the forces involved. It is obvious that for an adequate quantitative description of an activity such as walking, both kinetic and kinematic data are needed.

Work, energy and power

One of the remarkable features of normal gait is how energy is conserved by means of a number of optimisations. Abnormal gait patterns involve a loss of these optimisations, which may result in excessive energy expenditure and hence fatigue. The measurement, during walking, of energy transfers at individual joints and overall energy consumption is an important component of scientific gait analysis.

There is a subtle difference in viewpoint between the physical scientist and the biologist as far as work, energy and power are concerned. To the physical scientist, work is done when a force moves an object a certain distance. It is calculated as the product of the force and the distance; if a force of 2 N moves an object 3 m, the work done is:

$$2 \text{ N} \times 3 \text{ m} = 6 \text{ J (joules)}$$

The *joule* could also be called a newton-metre, but this would cause confusion with the identically named unit which is used to measure moment of force. *Energy* is the capacity to do work and is also measured in joules. It exists in two basic forms: *potential* or stored energy and *kinetic* or movement energy. In walking, there are alternating transfers between potential and kinetic energy, which will be described in Chapter 2. Power is the rate at which work is done; a rate of 1 J/s is a *watt*, which is familiar to users of electrical appliances.

The reason biologists regard these matters slightly differently from physical scientists is that muscles can use energy without shortening, in other words without doing any physical work. The potential energy stored in the muscles, in the form of ATP, is converted to mechanical energy in response to the muscle action potential. This energy is still used, even in an eccentric contraction, where the muscle actually gets longer while developing a force, which in physical terms is negative work. In other words, while everyone agrees that walking uphill involves the doing of work, the physicist might expect someone walking downhill to gain energy, whereas in reality the muscles are still activated and metabolic energy is still consumed. Even if a muscle shortens as it contracts, in a concentric contraction, the conversion of metabolic energy to mechanical energy is relatively inefficient, with a typical efficiency of around 25%. The old unit for measuring metabolic energy was the Calorie (the capital C indicating 1000 calories or 1 kilocalorie); the conversion factor is 4200 J or 4.2 kJ equals 1 Calorie (see Appendix 2).

The calculation of the mechanical power generated at joints has become an important part of the biomechanical study of gait. In a rotary movement, when a joint flexes or extends, the power is calculated as the product of the moment of force and the angular velocity, omega (ω):

$$P \text{ (watts)} = M \text{ (newton-metres)} \times \omega \text{ (radians per second)}$$

In Chapter 2, reference will be made to the power exchanges across the hip, knee and ankle joints at different stages of the gait cycle. When a muscle is contracting concentrically (e.g. a flexor muscle contracts while a joint is flexing), power is generated. If a muscle contracts eccentrically (e.g. a flexor muscle contracts while a joint is extending), it absorbs power. If a muscle contracts isometrically (e.g. a flexor muscle contracts while the joint angle is unchanging), no power exchange takes place. Although, in the gait cycle, power generation and absorption are often due to muscle contraction, it is important to realise that the stretching of ligaments and other soft tissues also involves power exchange. If a ligament is stretched, it absorbs power, with a resulting storage of potential energy. Some or all of this stored energy may be released later, with a resulting power generation.

In gait analysis, it is common practice to 'normalise' joint power by dividing it by body mass, giving a unit of watts per kilogram, in a similar way to the treatment of joint moments (mentioned above).

Worked example

When an individual who is pain and pathology free walks, the position of the ground reaction force in relation to the knee causes a muscular response. One common gait problem is that of crouch gait which can affect several different patient groups including people with cerebral palsy. By considering the mechanics involved we are able to estimate the moments and power about the knee and the forces in the quadriceps muscles in both these conditions.

To find the moments about the knee we need to know the perpendicular distance between the ground reaction force and the knee joint and the magnitude of the ground reaction force. Figure 1.23 shows a point during loading of the front foot. In both cases the ground reaction force was 500 N. The individual who is pain and pathology free had a distance to the knee of 0.08 m and the individual with crouch gait had a distance of 0.2 m. The moment may be found by multiplying the force by the perpendicular distance. Therefore the moments will be:

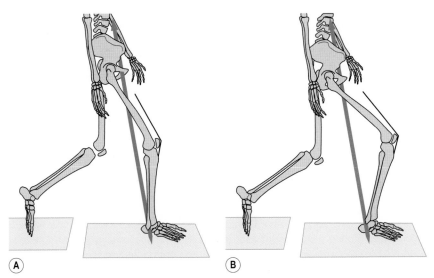

(A) (B)

Fig. 1.23 • Ground reaction forces in (A) normal gait and (B) crouch gait.

Moment for pain and pathology-free individual
$= 500 \times 0.08 = 40$ N·m
Moment for individual with crouch gait
$= 500 \times 0.2 = 100$ N·m

To find the eccentric power we will need to know the angular velocity of the knee. If the pain and pathology-free individual has an angular velocity of 150° per second and the individual with crouch gait has an angular velocity of 40° per second, the eccentric power may be found by:

First converting degrees per second into radians per second

$$150° \text{ per second} = 150/57.296 = 2.62 \text{ radians per second}$$
$$80° \text{ per second} = 40/57.296 = 0.70 \text{ radians per second}$$

Then using:

Power = Moment × Angular velocity
Eccentric power moment for pain and pathology-free individual $= 40 \times 2.62 = 140.8$ Watts
Eccentric power moment for individual with crouch gait $= 100 \times 0.70 = 70.0$ Watts

To find the muscle force we will need to know the knee moment and the perpendicular distance the muscle acts away from the knee joint. If in both cases the quadriceps tendon is only 0.06 m in front of the knee, the forces in the quadriceps may be found by:

$M = $ Force in quadriceps $\times 0.06$
Force in quadriceps $= M/0.06$
Force in quadriceps for pain and pathology-free individual $= 40/0.06 = 666.7$ N or 1.3 times body weight
Force in quadriceps for individual with crouch gait $= 100/0.06 = 1666.7$ N or 3.3 times body weight

Clearly crouch gait changes the mechanics and loading patterns of the knee and surrounding structures. The flexed position of the knee produces a much greater moment in the individual with crouch gait, however, they do not have the same eccentric control leading to a lower eccentric power. The increased moment at the knee has to be supported by the quadriceps but this leads to a load in the knee over two and half times that of the pain and pathology-free individual.

References

Duysens, J., Van de Crommert, H.W.A.A., 1998. Neural control of locomotion; part 1: the central pattern generator from cats to humans. Gait Posture 7, 131–141.

Guyton, A.C., 2005. Textbook of Medical Physiology, Twelfth ed. WB Saunders, Philadelphia, PA.

Park, S., Krebs, D.E., Mann, W., 1999. Hip muscle co-contraction: evidence from concurrent in vivo pressure measurement and force estimation. Gait Posture 10, 211–222.

Perry, J., 1992. Gait Analysis: Normal and Pathological Function. Slack Incorporated, Thorofare, NJ.

Pierrynowski, M.R., Galea, V., 2001. Enhancing the ability of gait analyses to differentiate between groups: scaling gait data to body size. Gait Posture 13, 193–201.

Pollo, F.E., Jackson, R.W., Komdeur, P., et al., 2003. Measuring dynamic knee motion with an instrumented spatial linkage device. In: Gait and Clinical Movement Analysis Society. Eighth Annual Meeting, Wilmington, Delaware, USA, pp. 15–16.

Richards, J., 2008. Biomechanics in Clinic and Research. Churchill Livingstone, Oxford.

Stansfield, B.W., Hillman, S.J., Hazlewood, M.E., et al., 2003. Normalization of gait data in children. Gait Posture 17, 81–87.

Further reading

Standring, S. (Ed.), 2009. Gray's Anatomy. fortieth ed. Churchill Livingstone, Oxford.

Normal gait

2

Michael Whittle   David Levine   Jim Richards

In order to understand pathological gait, it is necessary first to understand normal gait, since this provides the standard against which the gait of a patient can be judged. However, there are two pitfalls which need to be borne in mind when using this approach. Firstly, the term 'normal' covers both sexes, a wide range of ages and an even wider range of extremes of body geometry, so that an appropriate 'normal' standard needs to be chosen for the individual who is being studied. If results from an elderly female patient are compared with normal data obtained from physically fit young men, there will undoubtedly be large differences, whereas comparison with data from healthy elderly women may show the patient's gait to be well within normal limits which are appropriate to her sex and age. The second pitfall is that even though a patient's gait differs in some way from normal, it does not follow that this is in any way undesirable or that efforts should be made to turn it into a 'normal' gait. Many gait abnormalities are a compensation for some problem experienced by the patient and, although abnormal, they are nonetheless useful.

Having said all that, it is very important to understand normal gait and the terminology which is used to describe it, before going on to look at pathological gait. The chapter starts with a very brief historical review and then gives an overview of the gait cycle, before going on to study in detail how the different parts of the locomotor system are used in walking.

Walking and gait

As walking is such a familiar activity, it is difficult to define it without sounding pompous. However, it would be remiss not to attempt a definition. Normal human walking and running can be defined as 'a method of locomotion involving the use of the two legs, alternately, to provide both support and propulsion'. In order to exclude running, we must add 'at least one foot being in contact with the ground at all times'. Unfortunately, this definition excludes some forms of pathological gait which are generally regarded as being forms of walking, such as the 'three-point step-through gait' (see Fig. 3.21), in which there is an alternate use of two crutches and either one or two legs. It is probably both unreasonable and pointless to attempt a definition of walking which will apply to all cases – at least in a single sentence!

Gait is no easier to define than walking, many dictionaries regarding it as a word primarily for use in connection with horses! This is understandable, since quadruped animals have a repertoire of natural gaits (walking, trotting, cantering, galloping, etc.), as well as some artificial ones, such as that learned by 'Tennessee Walking Horses' in the area where one of the authors lives. Most people tend to use the words gait and walking interchangeably. However, there is a difference: the word gait describes 'the manner or style of walking', rather than the walking process itself. It thus makes more sense to talk about a difference in gait between two individuals than about a difference in walking.

History

The history of gait analysis has shown a steady progression from early descriptive studies, through increasingly sophisticated methods of measurement, to mathematical analysis and mathematical modelling. Only a brief account of the development of the discipline will be given here. Good reviews of the early years of gait analysis have been given by Garrison (1929), Bresler and Frankel (1950) and Steindler (1953). The more recent history of gait analysis, and of clinical gait analysis in particular, was covered in three excellent review papers by Sutherland (2001, 2002, 2005).

Descriptive studies

Walking has undoubtedly been observed ever since the time of the first men, but the systematic study of gait appears to date from the Renaissance when Leonardo da Vinci, Galileo and Newton all gave useful descriptions of walking. The earliest account using a truly scientific approach was in the classic *De Motu Animalum*, published in 1682 by Borelli, who worked in Italy and was a student of Galileo. Borelli measured the centre of gravity of the body and described how balance is maintained in walking by constant forward movement of the supporting area provided by the feet. The Weber brothers in Germany gave the first clear description of the gait cycle in 1836. They made accurate measurements of the timing of gait and of the pendulum-like swinging of the leg of a cadaver.

Kinematics

Two pioneers of kinematic measurement worked on opposite sides of the Atlantic in the 1870s. Marey, working in Paris, published a study of human limb movements in 1873. He made multiple photographic exposures, on a single plate, of a subject who was dressed in black, except for brightly illuminated stripes on the limbs. He also investigated the path of the centre of gravity of the body and the pressure beneath the foot. Eadweard Muybridge (born in England as Edward Muggeridge) became famous in California in 1878 by demonstrating that, when a horse is trotting, there are times when it has all four of its feet off the ground at once. The measurements were made using 24 cameras, triggered in quick succession as the horse ran into thin wires stretched across the track. In the next few years, Muybridge made a further series of studies, of naked human beings walking, running and performing a surprising variety of other activities!

The most serious application of the science of mechanics to human gait during the nineteenth century was the publication in Germany, in 1895, of *Der Gang des Menschen*, by Braune and Fischer. They employed a technique similar to Marey's, but using fluorescent strip-lights on the limbs instead of white stripes. The resulting photographs were used to determine the three-dimensional trajectories, velocities and accelerations of the body segments. Knowing the masses and accelerations of the body segments, they were then able to estimate the forces involved at all stages during the walking cycle.

Further valuable work on the dynamics of locomotion was done by Bernstein in Moscow in the 1930s. He developed a variety of photographic techniques for kinematic measurement and studied over 150 subjects. Particular attention was paid to the centre of gravity of the individual limb segments and of the body as a whole.

Force platforms

Further progress followed the development of the force platform (also called the forceplate). This instrument has contributed greatly to the scientific study of gait and is now standard equipment in gait laboratories. It measures the direction and magnitude of the ground reaction force beneath the foot. An early design was described by Amar in 1924 and an improved one by Elftman in 1938. Both were purely mechanical, the force applied to the platform causing the movement of a pointer. In Elftman's design the pointers were photographed by a high-speed movie camera.

Muscle activity

For a full understanding of normal gait, it is necessary to know which muscles are active during the different parts of the gait cycle. The role of the muscles was studied by Scherb, in Switzerland, during the 1940s, initially by palpating the muscles as his subject walked on a treadmill, then later by the use of electromyography (EMG). Further advances in the understanding of muscle activity and many other aspects of normal gait were made during the 1940s and 1950s by a very active group working in the University of California at San Francisco and Berkeley, notable among whom was Verne Inman. This group later went on to write *Human Walking* (Inman et al., 1981), published just after Inman's death, which to many people is the definitive textbook on normal gait. This has now gone through several editions, the latest edition of this being Rose and Gamble (2005). Another classic text on EMG is *Muscles Alive: Their Functions Revealed by Electromyography* by John Basmajian, which unfortunately has not been updated since 1985.

The use of EMG in gait analysis has received much attention but perhaps the most influential paper published was 'The use of surface electromyography in biomechanics' by Carlo De Luca in 1997, which gave a summary of recommendations but perhaps more importantly a summary of problems which at the time needed resolution. Further standardisation was achieved through the SENIAM (Surface Electro-MyoGraphy for the Non-Invasive Assessment of Muscles) project coordinated and managed by Hermie Hermens and Bart Freriks from Enschede, which is now considered by many as the definitive recommendations for electrode configuration and sensor positioning on specific muscles.

Mechanical analysis

A major contribution to the mechanical analysis of walking, also from the Californian group, was made by Bresler and Frankel (1950). They performed free-body calculations for the hip, knee and ankle joints, allowing for ground reaction forces, the effects of gravity on the limb segments and the inertial forces. The analytical techniques developed by these workers formed the basis of many current methods of modelling and analysis.

An important paper describing the possible mechanisms which the body uses to minimise energy consumption in walking, again from California, was published by Saunders et al. (1953). Further important work on energy consumption and in particular the energy transfers between the body segments in walking, was published by Cavagna and Margaria (1966), working in Italy. By 1960, research began to concentrate on the variability of walking, the development of gait in children and the deterioration of gait in old age. Patricia Murray, working in Milwaukee, Wisconsin, published a series of papers on these subjects, including a detailed review (Murray, 1967).

Mathematical modelling

Once the motions of the body segments and the actions of the different muscles had been examined and documented, attention passed to the forces generated across the joints. Although limited calculations

of this type had been made previously, the study by Paul (1965) was the first detailed analysis of hip joint forces during walking. A subsequent paper by the same author also included an analysis of the forces in the knee (Paul, 1966). Since then there have been many mathematical studies of force generation and transmission across the hip, knee and ankle.

The 1970s and 1980s saw great improvements in methods of measurement. The development of more convenient kinematic systems, based on electronics rather than photography, meant that results could be produced in minutes rather than days. Reliable force platforms with a high-frequency response became available, as well as convenient and reliable EMG systems. The availability of high-quality three-dimensional data on the kinetics and kinematics of walking, and the ease of access to powerful computers, made it possible to develop increasingly sophisticated mathematical models. Gait laboratories now routinely measure joint moments and powers for the hip, knee and ankle. Somewhat less reliably, estimates can also be made of muscle, ligament and joint contact forces.

The 1990s and 2000s have seen the emergence of increasingly powerful systems, higher speed cameras, greater portability, smaller markers and a wide variety of marker sets, and larger volumes of area that data can be attained from.

Clinical application

From the earliest days, it has been the hope of most of those working in this field that gait measurements would be found useful in the management of patients with walking disorders. Many of the early workers made studies of people who walked with abnormal gait patterns and some (notably Amar, Scherb and the Californian group) attempted to use the results for the benefit of individual patients. However, the results were not particularly impressive.

Since 1960, there has been a more serious attempt to take gait analysis out of the research laboratory and into the clinic. With the improvements in measurement and analytical techniques, the major limitation now is not the ability to produce high-quality data but knowing how best to use these data for the benefit of patients. It is fair to say that in the early days, far more progress was made in scientific gait analysis, particularly as applied to normal subjects, than in the application of these techniques for the benefit of those with gait disorders. However, since about

1980, there has been a steady increase in the effective use of gait analysis in the clinical management of patients.

As well as a gradual increase in the clinical use of scientific gait analysis, there has also been a growing interest in the use of observational or visual gait analysis. This has become much easier to perform since digital video cameras have become widely available, which is reviewed in more detail by Sutherland (2001, 2002, 2005).

Terminology used in gait analysis

The *gait cycle* is defined as the time interval between two successive occurrences of one of the repetitive events of walking. Although any event could be chosen to define the gait cycle, it is generally convenient to use the instant at which one foot contacts the ground ('initial contact'). If it is decided to start with initial contact of the right foot, as shown in Figure 2.1, then the cycle will continue until the right foot contacts the ground again. The left foot, of course, goes through exactly the same series of events as the right, but displaced in time by half a cycle.

The following terms are used to identify major events during the gait cycle:

1. Initial contact
2. Opposite toe off
3. Heel rise
4. Opposite initial contact
5. Toe off
6. Feet adjacent
7. Tibia vertical

These **seven events** subdivide the gait cycle into **seven periods,** four of which occur in the stance phase, when the foot is on the ground, and three in the swing phase, when the foot is moving forward through the air (Fig. 2.1). The stance phase, which is also called the 'support phase' or 'contact phase', lasts from initial contact to toe off. It is subdivided into:

1. Loading response
2. Mid-stance
3. Terminal stance
4. Pre-swing

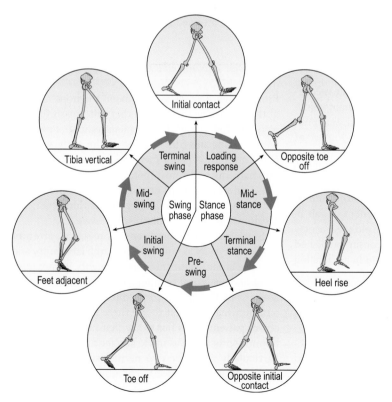

Fig. 2.1 • Positions of the legs during a single gait cycle by the right leg (green leg).

The swing phase lasts from toe off to the next initial contact. It is subdivided into:

1. Initial swing
2. Mid-swing
3. Terminal swing

The duration of a complete gait cycle is known as the *cycle time*, which is divided into *stance time* and *swing time*. Unfortunately, the nomenclature used to describe the gait cycle varies considerably from one publication to another. The present text attempts to use terms which will be understood by most people working in the field; alternative terminology will be given where appropriate. Wall et al. (1987) pointed out that the usual terminology is inadequate to describe some severely pathological gaits.

Gait cycle timing

Figure 2.2 shows the timings of initial contact and toe off for both feet during a little more than one gait cycle. Right initial contact occurs while the left foot is still on the ground and there is a period of *double support* (also known as 'double limb stance') between initial contact on the right and toe off on the left. During the swing phase on the left side, only the right foot is on the ground, giving a period of *right single support* (or 'single limb stance'), which ends with initial contact by the left foot. There is then another period of double support, until toe off on the right side. *Left single support* corresponds to the right swing phase and the cycle ends with the next initial contact on the right.

In each double support phase, one foot is forward, having just landed on the ground, and the other one is backward, being just about to leave the ground. When it is necessary to distinguish between the two legs in the double support phase, the leg in front is usually known as the 'leading' leg and the leg behind as the 'trailing' leg. The leading leg is in 'loading response', sometimes referred to as 'braking double support', 'initial double support' or 'weight acceptance'. The trailing leg is in 'pre-swing', also known as 'second', 'terminal' or 'thrusting' double support or 'weight release'.

In each gait cycle, there are thus two periods of double support and two periods of single support. The stance phase usually lasts about 60% of the cycle, the swing phase about 40% and each period of double support about 10%. However, this varies with the speed of walking, the swing phase becoming proportionally longer and the stance phase and double support phases shorter, as the speed increases (Murray, 1967). The final disappearance of the double support phase marks the transition from walking to running. Between successive steps in running there is a *flight phase*, also known as the 'float', 'double-float' or 'non-support' phase, when neither foot is on the ground. A detailed study of gait cycle timing was published by Blanc et al. (1999).

Foot placement

The terms used to describe the placement of the feet on the ground are shown in Figure 2.3. The *stride length* is the distance between two successive placements of the same foot. It consists of two step lengths, left and right, each of which is the distance by which the named foot moves forward in front of the other one. In pathological gait, it is common

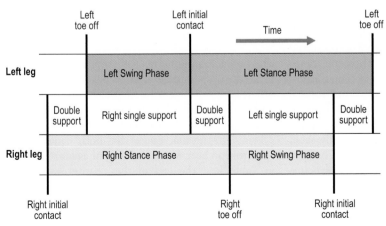

Fig. 2.2 • Timing of single and double support during a little more than one gait cycle, starting with right initial contact.

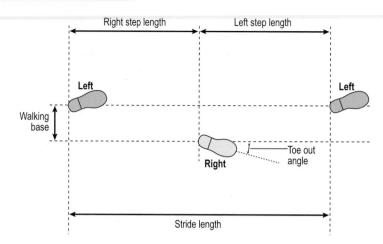

Fig. 2.3 • Terms used to describe foot placement on the ground.

for the two *step lengths* to be different. If the left foot is moved forward to take a step and the right one is brought up beside it, rather than in front of it, the right step length will be zero. It is even possible for the step length on one side to be negative, for example, if the left foot never catches up with the right foot, the distance between the left and right feet will be negative. However, the *stride* length starting with the left heel strike must always be the same as the stride length starting with the right heelstrike, unless the subject is walking around a curve where the inside leg will have a shorter stride length than the outside leg. This definition of a 'stride', consisting of one 'step' by each foot, breaks down in some pathological gaits, in which one foot makes a series of 'hopping' movements while the other is in the air (Wall et al., 1987). There is no satisfactory nomenclature to deal with this situation.

The *walking base* (also known as the 'stride width' or 'base of support') is the side-to-side distance between the line of the two feet, usually measured at the midpoint of the back of the heel but sometimes below the centre of the ankle joint. The preferred unit for stride length and step length is the metre and for the walking base, millimetres. The pattern of walking known as 'tandem gait' involves walking with the heel of one foot placed directly in front of the toes of the other, i.e. with a walking base close to zero. Although this pattern is not typically seen, even as a pathological gait, it requires good balance and coordination and it is often used by the police as a test for intoxication!

The *toe out* (or, less commonly, *toe in*) is the angle in degrees between the direction of progression and a reference line on the sole of the foot. The reference line varies from one study to another; it may be defined anatomically but is commonly the midline of the foot, as judged by eye.

It is common experience that you need to walk more carefully on ice than on asphalt. Whether or not the foot slips during walking depends on two things: the coefficient of friction between the foot and the ground, and the relationship between the vertical force and the forces parallel to the walking surface (front-to-back and side-to-side). The ratio of the horizontal to the vertical force is known as the 'utilised coefficient of friction' and slippage will occur if this exceeds the actual coefficient of friction between the foot and the ground. In normal walking, a coefficient of friction of 0.35–0.40 is generally sufficient to prevent slippage; the most hazardous part of the gait cycle for slippage is initial contact. There is a fairly extensive literature on foot-to-ground friction and slippage, e.g. Cham and Redfern (2002) and Burnfield et al. (2005).

Cadence, cycle time and speed

The *cadence* is the number of steps taken in a given time, the usual unit being steps per minute. In most other types of scientific measurement, complete cycles are counted, but as there are two steps in a single gait cycle, the cadence is a measure of half-cycles. The normal ranges for both cadence and *cycle time* in both sexes at different ages are showed in Table 1 at the end of this chapter, where we consider the effect of age in more detail.

The *speed* of walking is the distance covered by the whole body in a given time. It should be measured in metres per second. Many authors use the term 'velocity' in place of 'speed' but this is an incorrect usage of the term, unless the direction of walking is also stated, since velocity is a vector. The instantaneous speed varies from one instant to another during the walking cycle, but the average speed is the product of the cadence and the stride length, providing appropriate units are used. The cadence, in steps per minute, corresponds to half-strides per 60 seconds or full strides per 120 seconds. The speed can thus be calculated from cadence and stride length using the formula:

$$\text{speed (m/s)} = \text{stride length (m)} \times \text{cadence(steps/min)}/120$$

If cycle time is used in place of cadence, the calculation becomes much more straightforward:

$$\text{speed (m/s)} = \text{stride length (m)}/\text{cycle time (s)}$$

The walking speed thus depends on the two step lengths, which in turn depend to a large extent on the duration of the swing phase on each side. The step length is the amount by which the foot can be moved forwards during the swing phase, so that a short swing phase on one side will generally reduce the step length on that side. If the foot catches on the ground, this may terminate the swing phase and thereby further reduce both step length and walking speed. In pathological gait, the step length is often shortened, but it behaves in a way which is counterintuitive. When pathology affects one foot more than the other, an individual will usually try to spend a shorter time on the 'bad' foot and correspondingly longer on the 'good' one. Shortening the stance phase on the 'bad' foot means bringing the 'good' foot to the ground sooner, thereby shortening both the duration of the swing phase and the step length on that side. Thus, a short step length on

one side generally means problems with single support on the *other* side.

When making comparisons between individuals, particularly with children, it is useful to allow for differences in size. This is done by dividing a measurement by some aspect of body size, such as height (stature) or leg length, a procedure generally known as 'normalisation'. It is thus fairly common to see walking speed expressed in 'statures per second' or to see measures such as 'step factor', which is step length divided by leg length (Sutherland, 1997).

Since walking speed depends on both cadence and stride length, it follows that speed may be changed by altering only one of these variables, for instance by increasing the cadence while keeping the stride length constant. In practice, however, people normally change their walking speed by adjusting both cadence and stride length. Sekiya and Nagasaki (1998) defined the 'walk ratio' as step length (m) divided by step rate (steps/min) and found that it was fairly constant in both males and females over a range of walking speeds from very slow to very fast. Macellari et al. (1999) made a detailed study of the relationships between gender, body size, walking speed, gait timing and foot placement.

Outline of the gait cycle

The purpose of this section is to provide the reader with an overview of the gait cycle, to make the detailed description which follows a little easier to follow. The cycle is illustrated by Figures 2.4 and 2.10–2.18, all of which are taken from a single walk

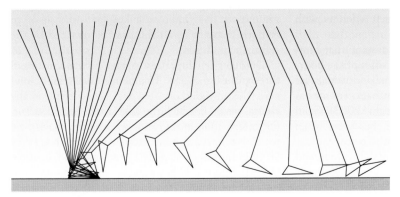

Fig. 2.4 • Position of the right leg in the sagittal plane at 40 ms intervals during a single gait cycle.

by a 22-year-old normal female, weight 540 N (55 kg, 121 lb), walking barefoot with a cycle time of 0.88 s (cadence 136 steps/min), a stride length of 1.50 m and a speed of 1.70 m/s. The individual measurements from this subject do not always correspond to 'average' values, because of the normal variability between individuals, although they are all close to the normal range. The measurements were all made in the plane of progression, which is a vertical plane aligned to the direction of the walk; in normal walking it closely corresponds to the sagittal plane of the body. The data were obtained using a Vicon motion system and a Bertec force platform. It should be noted that different laboratories use different methods of measurement, so that other publications may quote different values for some of the measured variables. The reader should thus concentrate on the changes in the variables during the gait cycle, rather than on their absolute values.

When examining diagrams of the joint angles through the gait cycle, it is essential to understand how the angles are defined. Generally speaking, the knee angle is defined as the angle between the femur and the tibia and there is usually no ambiguity. The ankle angle is usually defined as the angle between the tibia and an arbitrary line in the foot. Although this angle is normally around 90°, it is conventional to define it as 0°, dorsiflexion and plantarflexion being movements in the positive and negative directions. In this book, dorsiflexion is a positive angle, but in some other publications it is negative. The 'hip' angle may be measured in two different ways: the angle between the vertical and the femur, and the angle between the pelvis and the femur. The latter is the 'true' hip angle and is usually defined so that 0° is close to the hip angle in the standing position. Forward flexion of the trunk appears as hip flexion when the hip angle is defined with reference to the pelvis, but not when it is defined with reference to the vertical.

The descriptions which follow assume that symmetry is present between the two sides of the body. This is approximately true for normal individuals, although detailed examination shows that everyone has some degree of asymmetry (Sadeghi, 2003). Such subtle asymmetries are negligible, however, when contrasted with the majority of pathological gaits.

Some gait studies are performed barefoot and some with the subject wearing shoes. Oeffinger et al. (1999) found small differences in some of the gait parameters between these two conditions

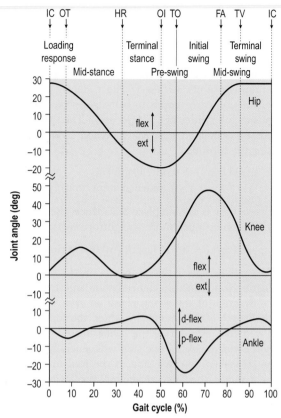

Fig. 2.5 • Sagittal plane joint angles (degrees) during a single gait cycle of right hip (flexion positive), knee (flexion positive) and ankle (dorsiflexion positive). IC = initial contact; OT = opposite toe off; HR = heel rise; OI = opposite initial contact; TO = toe off; FA = feet adjacent; TV = tibia vertical.

in children, but did not consider them to be clinically significant. It is usually at the discretion of the investigator whether or not shoes are worn, although in some cases (e.g. when an ankle–foot orthosis or an orthotic insole is used) this may be dictated by the subject's condition.

During gait, important movements occur in all three planes – sagittal, frontal and transverse. However, this introductory text will concentrate on the sagittal plane, in which the largest movements occur. For information on the motion in other planes, the reader is referred to more detailed texts, such as Perry (1992), Inman et al. (1981) or Rose and Gamble (1994). Figure 2.4 shows the successive positions of the right leg at 40 ms intervals, measured over a single gait cycle. Figure 2.5 shows the corresponding sagittal

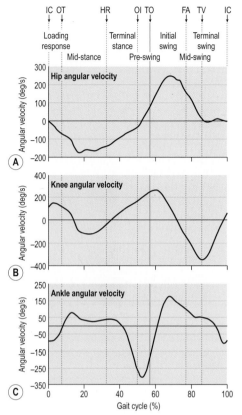

Fig. 2.6 (A–C) • Sagittal plane joint angular velocities during a single gait cycle.

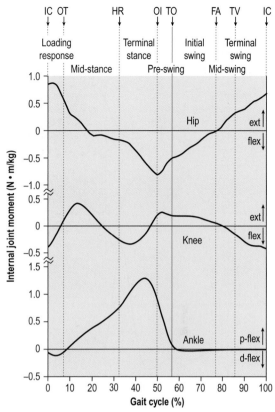

Fig. 2.7 • Sagittal plane internal joint moments (newton-metres per kilogram body mass) during a single gait cycle of right hip (extensor moment positive), knee (extensor moment positive) and ankle (plantarflexor moment positive). Abbreviations as in Figure 2.5.

plane angles at the hip, knee and ankle joints and Figure 2.6 shows the sagittal plane angular velocity of the hip, knee and ankle joints.

Figure 2.7 shows the internal joint moments (in newton-metres per kilogram body mass) and Figure 2.8 the joint powers (in watts per kilogram body mass). Different authors have used different units for the measurement of moments and powers; those used here are scaled for body mass, but not for the length of the limb segments. In Figure 2.8, the annotations H1–H3, K1–K4 and A1–A2 refer to the peaks of power absorption and generation described by Winter (1991).

Figure 2.9 shows a 'butterfly diagram', described by Pedotti (1977). This is a plot of the ground reaction vectors and is made up of successive representations, at 10 ms intervals, of the magnitude, direction and point of application of the ground reaction force vector. The vectors move across the diagram from left to right and create a shape that resembles the wings of a butterfly.

Figure 2.10 gives the typical activity of a number of key muscles or muscle groups during the gait cycle. It is based largely on data from Perry (1992), Inman et al. (1981) and Rose and Gamble (1994). Similar, though not identical, data for these and other muscles were given by Sutherland (1984) and Winter (1991). Although Figure 2.10 shows a typical pattern, it is not the only possible one. One of the interesting things about gait is the way in which the same movement may be achieved in a number of different ways and this particularly applies to the use of muscles, so that two people may walk with the same 'normal' gait pattern but using different combinations of muscles. The pattern of muscle usage not only varies from one subject to another but it is also affected by fatigue and varies with walking speed, in a single person. The muscular system is said to possess

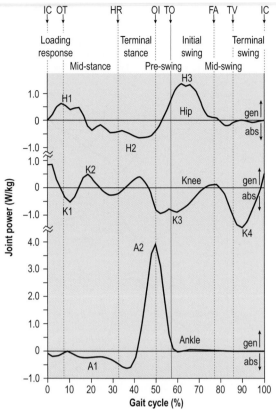

Fig. 2.8 • Sagittal plane joint powers (watts per kilogram body mass) during a single gait cycle of right hip, knee and ankle. Power generation is positive, absorption is negative. See text for meaning of H1, H2, etc. Other abbreviations as in Figure 2.5.

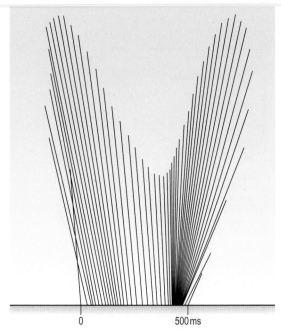

Fig. 2.9 • 'Butterfly diagram' representation of ground reaction force vector at 10 ms intervals. Progression is from left to right.

'redundancy', which means that if a particular muscle cannot be used, its functions may be taken over another muscle or group of muscles. A good review of muscle activity in gait was provided by Shiavi (1985).

Figures 2.11–2.19 show the positions of the two legs and the ground reaction force vector beneath the right foot (where present), at the seven major events of the gait cycle and at two additional points – near the beginning of the loading response (Fig. 2.12) and halfway through mid-stance (Fig. 2.14). The description is based on a gait cycle from right initial contact to the next right initial contact. However, the gait cycle could just as easily have been defined using the left leg.

Throughout the text, references will be made to the position of the ground reaction force vector relative to the axis of a joint and to the resulting joint moments. This approach, known as 'vector projection', is an approximation at best, since it neglects the mass of the leg below the joint in question (especially important at the hip) and also ignores the acceleration and deceleration of the limb segments (which primarily lead to errors in the swing phase). However, the author has used this approach since it makes it much easier to understand joint moments. The graphs for joint moments (Fig. 2.7) and joint powers (Fig. 2.8) were calculated 'correctly', using a method known as 'inverse dynamics', which is based on the kinematics, the ground reaction force and the subject's anthropometry. Wells (1981) discussed the relative merits of these two methods for estimating joint moments.

Upper body

The upper body moves forwards throughout the gait cycle. Its speed varies a little, being fastest during the double support phases and slowest in the middle of the stance and swing phases. The trunk twists about a vertical axis, the shoulder girdle rotating in the opposite direction to the pelvis. The arms swing out of phase with the legs, so that the left leg and the left side of the pelvis move forwards at the same time as the right arm and the right side of the shoulder girdle. Lamoth et al. (2002) made a detailed study of

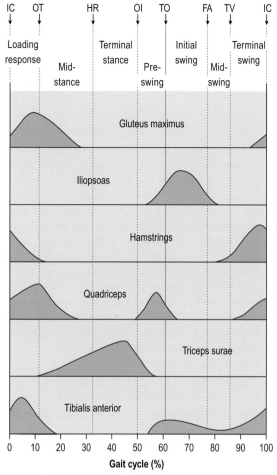

IC OT   HR   OI TO   FA TV   IC

Loading   Terminal   Initial   Terminal
response   stance   swing   swing
        Mid-   Pre-   Mid-
        stance   swing   swing

Gluteus maximus

Iliopsoas

Hamstrings

Quadriceps

Triceps surae

Tibialis anterior

0   10   20   30   40   50   60   70   80   90   100
Gait cycle (%)

Fig. 2.10 • Typical activity of major muscle groups during the gait cycle. Abbreviations as in Figure 2.5. The timings of the events of the gait cycle are typical and not derived from a single subject.

the relative motion between the pelvis and the trunk at different walking speeds. Murray (1967) found average total excursions of 7° for the shoulder girdle and 12° for the pelvis, in adult males walking at free speed. The fluidity and efficiency of walking depend to some extent on the motions of the trunk and arms, but these movements are commonly ignored in clinical gait analysis and have been relatively neglected in gait research. The whole trunk rises and falls twice during the cycle, through a total range of about 46 mm (Perry, 1992), being lowest during double support and highest in the middle of the stance and swing phases. An approximation to this vertical motion can be seen in the position of the hip joint in Figure 2.4. The trunk also moves from side to side,

once in each cycle, the trunk being over each leg during its stance phase, as might be expected from the need for support. The total range of side-to-side movement is also about 46 mm (Perry, 1992). The pelvis, as well as twisting about a vertical axis, also tips slightly, both backwards and forwards (with an associated change in lumbar lordosis) and from side to side. The spinal muscles are selectively activated so that the head moves less than the pelvis, which is important for providing a stable platform for vision (Prince et al., 1994).

Hip

The hip flexes and extends once during the cycle (Fig. 2.5). The limit of flexion is reached around the middle of the swing phase and the hip is then kept flexed until initial contact. The peak extension is reached before the end of the stance phase, after which the hip begins to flex again.

Knee

The knee shows two flexion and two extension peaks during each gait cycle. It is more or less fully extended before initial contact, flexes during the loading response and the early part of mid-stance ('stance phase knee flexion'), extends again during the later part of mid-stance, then starts flexing again, reaching a peak during initial swing ('swing phase knee flexion'). It extends again prior to the next initial contact.

Ankle and foot

The ankle is usually within a few degrees of the neutral position for dorsiflexion/plantarflexion at the time of initial contact. After initial contact, the ankle plantarflexes, bringing the forefoot down onto the ground. During mid-stance, the tibia moves forward over the foot, and the ankle joint becomes dorsiflexed. Before opposite initial contact, the ankle angle again changes, a major plantarflexion taking place until just after toe off. During the swing phase, the ankle moves back into dorsiflexion until the forefoot has cleared the ground (around feet adjacent), after which something close to the neutral position is maintained until the next initial contact. In the frontal plane, the foot is slightly inverted (supinated, adducted or varus) at initial contact. The foot pronates as it contacts the ground, then moves back into supination as the ankle angle changes from plantarflexion to dorsiflexion, this supinated attitude being maintained as the heel rises and the ankle plantarflexes prior to toe off. Some degree of supination is retained throughout the swing phase.

The gait cycle in detail

Each of the following sections begins with some general remarks about the events surrounding a particular event in the gait cycle and then describes what is happening in the upper body, hips, knees, ankles and feet, with particular reference to the activity of the muscles. These sections are very detailed and may be too much to comprehend in one 'pass'. It is suggested that the reader should skip the moments and powers on the first reading, but should go back to them later, to gain a deeper understanding of the mechanical processes underlying the gait cycle. The figures shown in this section represent the normal positions of the lower limbs and pelvis at different events during gait and the ground reaction force vector expected.

More detailed descriptions of the events of normal gait are given by Murray (1967), Perry (1992), Inman et al. (1981) and Rose and Gamble (1994).

Initial contact (Fig. 2.11)

1. General: Initial contact is the beginning of the loading response, which is the first period of the stance phase. Initial contact is frequently called 'heelstrike', since in normal individuals there is often a distinct impact between the heel and the ground,

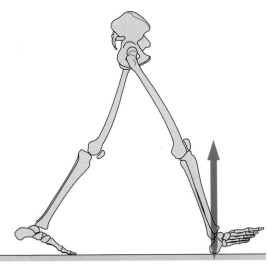

Fig. 2.11 • Initial contact: position of right leg (green), left leg (grey) and ground reaction force vector during the heelstrike transient. This illustration also applies to terminal foot contact.

known as the 'heelstrike transient'. Other names for this event are 'heel contact', 'footstrike' or 'foot contact'. The direction of the ground reaction force changes from generally upwards during the heelstrike transient (Fig. 2.11) to upwards and backwards in the loading response, immediately afterwards (Fig. 2.12). This change in direction can also be seen in the butterfly diagram (Fig. 2.9), where the force vector changes direction immediately after initial contact.

2. Upper body: The trunk is about half a stride length behind the leading (right) foot at the time of initial contact. In the side-to-side direction, the trunk is crossing the midline in its range of travel, moving towards the right, as the foot on that side makes contact. The trunk is twisted, the left shoulder and the right side of the pelvis each being at their furthest forwards and the left arm at its most advanced. The amount of arm swinging varies greatly from one person to another and it also increases with the speed of walking. At the time of initial contact, Murray (1967) found the mean elbow flexion was 8° and the shoulder flexion 45°.

3. Hip: The attitude of the legs at the time of initial contact is shown in Fig. 2.11. The maximum flexion of the hip (generally around 30°) is reached around the middle of the swing phase, after which it changes little until initial contact. The hamstrings are active during the latter part of the swing phase (since they act to prevent knee hyperextension); gluteus maximus begins to contract around the time of initial contact and together these muscles start the extension of the hip, which will be complete around the time of opposite initial contact (Fig. 2.5).

4. Knee: The knee extends rapidly at the end of the swing phase, becoming more or less straight just before initial contact and then starting to flex again (Figs 2.5 and 2.11). This extension is generally thought to be passive, although Perry (1992) states that it involves quadriceps contraction. Except in very slow walking, the hamstrings contract eccentrically at the end of the swing phase, to act as a braking mechanism to prevent knee hyperextension. This contraction continues into the beginning of the stance phase.

5. Ankle and foot: The ankle is generally close to its neutral position in plantarflexion/dorsiflexion at the time of initial contact. Since the tibia is sloping backwards, the foot slopes upwards and only the heel contacts the ground (Fig. 2.11). The foot is usually slightly supinated (inverted, adducted or varus) at this time and most people show a wear pattern on the lateral side of the heel of the shoe. Tibialis anterior is active throughout swing and in early stance, having maintained dorsiflexion during the swing phase and in preparation for the controlled movement into plantarflexion which occurs following initial contact.

6. Moments and powers: At the time of initial contact, there is an internal extensor moment at the hip (Fig. 2.7), produced by contraction of the hip extensors (gluteus maximus and the hamstrings, Fig. 2.10). As the hip joint moves in the direction of extension, these muscles contract concentrically and generate power (H1 in Fig. 2.8). The knee shows an internal flexor moment, due to contraction of the hamstrings (Fig. 2.10) as they prevent hyperextension at the end of the swing phase. As the knee starts to flex, concentric contraction of the hamstrings, as well as the release of energy stored in the ligaments of the extended knee, results in a short-lived power generation (unnamed peak in Fig. 2.8). Little moment or power exchange occurs at the ankle until just after initial contact. The 'heelstrike' involves an absorption of energy by the elastic tissues of the heel and by compliant materials in footwear, very little of which could be recovered later in the stance phase. The amount of energy lost to the environment as sound and heat in this way is probably fairly small.

Loading response (Fig. 2.12)

1. General: The loading response is the double support period between initial contact and opposite toe off. During this period, the foot is lowered to the ground by plantarflexion of the ankle. The ground reaction force increases rapidly in magnitude, its direction being upwards and backwards. In the subject used for illustration, loading response occupied the period from 0% to 7% of the cycle; this is unusually short, loading response typically occupying the first 10–12% of the cycle. Figure 2.12 represents 2% of the cycle.

2. Upper body: During loading response, the trunk is at its lowest vertical position, about 20 mm below its average level for the whole cycle; its instantaneous forward speed is at its greatest, around 10% higher than the average speed for the whole cycle. It continues to move laterally towards the right foot. The arms, having reached their maximum forward (left) and backward (right) positions, begin to return.

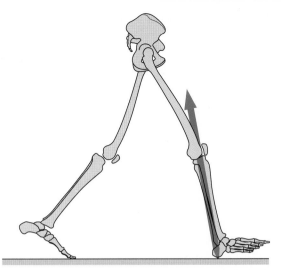

Fig. 2.12 • Loading response: position of right leg (green), left leg (grey) and ground reaction force vector 20 ms after initial contact.

3. Hip: During loading response, the hip begins to extend (Fig. 2.5), through concentric contraction of the hip extensors, gluteus maximus and the hamstrings (Fig. 2.10).

4. Knee: From its nearly fully extended position at initial contact, the knee flexes during loading response (Fig. 2.5), initiating the 'stance phase flexion'. This is accompanied by eccentric contraction of the quadriceps (Fig. 2.10), to limit the speed and magnitude of flexion.

5. Ankle and foot: The loading response period of the gait cycle, also called the 'initial rocker', 'heel rocker' or 'heel pivot', involves plantarflexion at the ankle (Fig. 2.5). The plantarflexion is controlled by eccentric contraction of the tibialis anterior muscle. The movement into plantarflexion is accompanied by pronation of the foot and internal rotation of the tibia, there being an automatic coupling between pronation/supination of the foot and internal/external rotation of the tibia (Inman et al., 1981; Rose and Gamble, 1994). The direction of the force vector changes from that shown in Figure 2.10 to that shown in Figure 2.12, within 10–20 ms.

6. Moments and powers: As described above (p. 46, Initial contact, section 6), the hip shows an internal extensor moment with power generation during the loading response and the knee shows an internal flexor moment with power generation. At the ankle, the posterior placement of the force vector

(Fig. 2.12) produces an external plantarflexor moment. In the normal individual, this is resisted by an internal dorsiflexor moment (Fig. 2.7) produced by tibialis anterior (Fig. 2.10), which contracts eccentrically, absorbing power (Fig. 2.8) and permitting the foot to be lowered gently to the ground. Should tibialis anterior fail to generate sufficient moment, the foot plantarflexes too rapidly, producing an audible 'foot slap'.

Opposite toe off (Fig. 2.13)

1. General: Opposite toe off, also known as 'opposite foot off', is the end of the double support period known as loading response and the beginning of mid-stance, the first period of single support. The forefoot, which was being lowered by plantarflexion of the ankle, contacts the ground at 'foot flat', also known as 'forefoot contact', which generally occurs around the time of opposite toe off. On the opposite (left) side, it marks the end of the stance phase and the beginning of the swing phase. In the subject used for illustration, opposite toe off (Fig. 2.13) occurred at 7% of the cycle and foot flat at 8% of the cycle.

2. Upper body: At opposite toe off, the left shoulder and arm, having reached their most advanced position, are now moving back again. Similarly, the pelvis

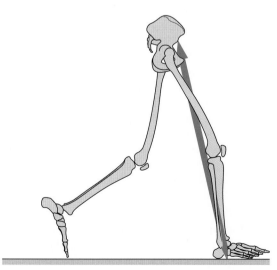

Fig. 2.13 • Opposite toe off: position of right leg (green), left leg (grey) and ground reaction force vector.

on the right side now starts to twist back towards the neutral position. The trunk, having reached its lowest position during loading response, now begins to gain height but to lose forward speed, as a result of the backward and upward direction of the ground reaction force, acting on the centre of gravity of the body. This represents a conversion of kinetic energy to potential energy, similar to that seen in a child's swing at its lowest point before it begins to climb up again.

3. Hip: The hip flexion angle is around 25° at time of opposite toe off (Fig. 2.5). The hip continues to extend, by concentric contraction of the gluteus maximus and hamstrings.

4. Knee: At opposite toe off, the knee is continuing to flex, reaching the peak of 'stance phase knee flexion' early in mid-stance, after which it begins to extend again (Fig. 2.5). The magnitude of the stance phase flexion is very sensitive to walking speed; it disappears in a very slow walk. Quadriceps contraction (eccentric then concentric) permits the knee to act like a spring, preventing the vertical force from building up too rapidly (Perry, 1974).

5. Ankle and foot: As soon as the foot is flat on the ground, around opposite toe off, the direction of ankle motion changes from plantarflexion to dorsiflexion, as the tibia moves over the now stationary foot (Fig. 2.5). Both foot pronation and internal tibial rotation reach a peak around opposite toe off and begin to reverse. These two motions are 'coupled', i.e. they always occur together, due in part to the geometry of the ankle and subtalar joints (Inman et al., 1981; Rose and Gamble, 1994). Tibialis anterior ceases to contract, to be replaced by contraction of the triceps surae (Fig. 2.10).

6. Moments and powers: At opposite toe off, the hip continues to have an internal extensor moment with power generation, as described above (p. 46, Initial contact, section 6). At the knee, the force vector lies behind the joint (Fig. 2.13), producing an external flexor moment. This is opposed by an internal extensor moment (Fig. 2.7), generated by the quadriceps muscles (Fig. 2.10). These contract eccentrically, absorbing power (K1 in Fig. 2.8). The line of the ground reaction force begins to move forwards along the foot (Fig. 2.13), causing the internal dorsiflexor moment at the ankle to become smaller and then to reverse, to become a plantarflexor moment (Fig. 2.7). Little power exchange occurs at the ankle at this time.

Mid-stance (Fig. 2.14)

1. General: Mid-stance is the period of the gait cycle between opposite toe off and heel rise, although the term has been used in the past to describe an event in the gait cycle when the swing phase leg passes the stance phase leg, corresponding to the swing phase event of 'feet adjacent', or the point in time when the anterior posterior component of the ground reaction force is zero. In the subject used for illustration, mid-stance occupied the period from 7% to 32% of the cycle; Figure 2.14A represents 18% of the cycle and Figure 2.14B the event when the anterior posterior reaction force is zero.

2. Upper body: The period of mid-stance sees the trunk climbing to its highest point, about 20 mm above the mean level, and slowing its forward speed, as the kinetic energy of forward motion is converted to the potential energy of height. The side-to-side motion of the trunk also reaches its peak during mid-stance, the trunk being displaced about 20 mm from its central position, towards the side of the stance (right) leg. Like the feet, the arms pass each other during mid-stance, as each follows the motion of the opposite leg. The twisting of the trunk has now disappeared, as both the shoulder girdle and pelvis pass through neutral before twisting the other way.

3. Hip: During the mid-stance period, the hip continues to extend, moving from a flexed attitude to an extended one (Fig. 2.5). Concentric contraction of gluteus maximus and the hamstrings ceases during this period, as hip extension is achieved by inertia and gravity. Throughout mid-stance and terminal stance, significant muscle activity about the hip joint takes place in the frontal plane. As soon as the opposite foot has left the ground, the pelvis is supported only by the stance phase hip. It is permitted to dip down slightly on the side of the swinging leg, but its position is maintained by contraction of the hip abductors, especially gluteus medius and tensor fascia lata.

4. Knee: During mid-stance, the knee reaches its peak of stance phase flexion and starts to extend again (Fig. 2.5), initially through concentric contraction of the quadriceps. The peak generally occurs between 15% and 20% of the gait cycle. Its magnitude is variable, both from one individual to another and with the speed of walking, but it is commonly between 10° and 20°.

5. Ankle and foot: The 'mid-stance rocker', also called the 'second rocker' or 'ankle rocker', occurs during mid-stance and terminal stance. It is characterised by forward rotation of the tibia about the ankle joint, as the foot remains flat on the floor, the ankle angle changing from plantarflexion to dorsiflexion, with the triceps surae contracting eccentrically. The actual angles vary with the method of measurement; most authors report larger angles than those seen in Figure 2.5. External rotation of the tibia and coupled supination of the foot occur during mid-stance and terminal stance. The ground reaction force vector moves forward along the foot from the time of foot flat onwards, moving into the forefoot prior to heel rise. The movement of the foot into supination peaks in mid-stance and then begins to reverse towards pronation.

6. Moments and powers: During mid-stance, the internal extensor moment at the hip, generated by contraction of the extensor muscles, declines and disappears, to be replaced by a moment in the opposite direction (Fig. 2.7). At the knee, the force vector remains behind the joint, producing an external flexor moment, opposed by an internal extensor moment (Fig. 2.7), due to quadriceps contraction (Fig. 2.10). According to Perry (1992), only the vasti,

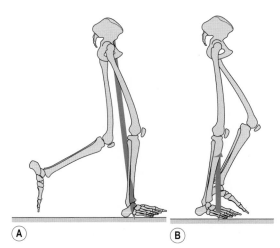

Fig. 2.14 • (A) Mid-stance: position of right leg (green), left leg (grey) and ground reaction force vector 100 ms after opposite toe off. (B) Mid-stance event when the anterior posterior component of the ground reaction force is zero.

and not the rectus femoris, are active at this time. As the direction of knee motion changes from flexion to extension (Fig. 2.5), power generation takes place (K2 in Fig. 2.8). The ankle shows an increasing internal plantarflexor moment throughout mid-stance and into terminal stance (Fig. 2.7), as the force vector moves into the forefoot. This moment is generated by the triceps surae (Fig. 2.10), contracting eccentrically and absorbing power (A1 in Fig. 2.8).

Heel rise (Fig. 2.15)

1. General: Heel rise, also called 'heel off', marks the transition from mid-stance to terminal stance. It is the time at which the heel begins to lift from the walking surface. Its timing varies considerably, both from one individual to another and with the speed of walking. The subject used for illustration showed heel rise at 32% of the gait cycle.

2. Upper body: By heel rise, the trunk is falling from its highest point, reached during mid-stance. The lateral displacement over the supporting (right) leg also begins to diminish, in preparation for the transfer of weight back to the left leg. As the right hip extends and the leg moves backwards, the right side of the pelvis twists backwards with it and the arm and shoulder girdle on the right move forwards.

3. Hip: At heel rise and into terminal stance, the hip continues to extend (Fig. 2.5). Peak hip extension is

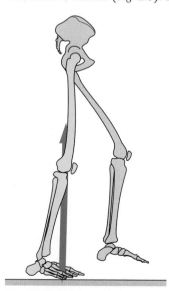

Fig. 2.15 • Heel rise: position of right leg (green), left leg (grey) and ground reaction force vector.

reached around the time of opposite initial contact. The activity of the hip abductors in the frontal plane is still required to stabilise the pelvis, although this activity ceases prior to initial contact by the other foot.

4. Knee: The knee has an extension peak close to the time of heel rise (Fig. 2.5). Around this time, active ankle plantarflexion brings the ground reaction force forward, moving it into the forefoot and in front of the knee joint (barely visible in Fig. 2.15). This attempts to extend the knee, an effect known as the 'plantarflexion/knee extension couple', which becomes very important in some pathological gaits. Contraction of the gastrocnemius augments the action of the soleus as far as the ankle joint is concerned, but it also acts as a flexor at the knee, preventing hyperextension and subsequently initiating knee flexion.

5. Ankle and foot: The peak of ankle dorsiflexion is reached some time after heel rise (Fig. 2.5). Triceps surae initially maintains the ankle angle as the knee begins to flex, with movement into plantarflexion only beginning late in terminal stance. The tibia becomes increasingly externally rotated and the foot becomes increasingly supinated, the two being linked through coupled motion at the subtalar joint. As the heel rises, the toes remain flat on the ground and extension occurs at the metatarsophalangeal (MTP) joints, along an oblique line across the foot, known as the 'metatarsal break' or 'toe break'. From the time that the heel rises, hindfoot inversion (adduction or varus angulation) is seen.

6. Moments and powers: At heel rise there is a small but increasing internal hip flexor moment (Fig. 2.7). The source of this internal flexor moment does not appear to have been fully explained in the literature, although it could be due to a combination of adductor longus and rectus femoris contraction and stretching of ligaments as the hip moves into extension, with a resulting power absorption (H2 in Fig. 2.8). At the knee, quadriceps contraction has ceased prior to heel rise and the internal knee moment has reversed to become flexor. According to Perry (1992), this occurs because the upper body moves forward faster than the tibia. If the ankle joint were totally free, the forward motion of the body would simply dorsiflex the ankle. However, contraction of the triceps surae (Fig. 2.10) slows down the forward motion of the tibia so that as the femur moves forwards, an external extensor moment is generated at the knee, opposed by an internal flexor moment (Fig. 2.7). Only small and variable power exchanges occur at the knee around heel rise. At the ankle, the internal plantarflexor moment continues to increase, as first the soleus and then both soleus and gastrocnemius together (triceps surae in Fig. 2.10) contract increasingly strongly. The contraction is initially eccentric, with power absorption (A1 in Fig. 2.8).

Opposite initial contact (Fig. 2.16)

1. General: As might be expected, opposite initial contact in symmetrical gait occurs at close to 50% of the cycle. It marks the end of the period of single support and the beginning of pre-swing, which is the second period of double support. At the time of opposite initial contact, also known as 'opposite foot contact', the hip begins to flex, the knee is already flexing and the ankle is plantarflexing. The period between heel rise and toe off (terminal stance followed by pre-swing) is sometimes called the 'terminal rocker'. This is appropriate, since the leg is now rotating forwards about the forefoot, rather than about the ankle joint. Another term for this period is the 'push off' phase. Perry (1974) objected to this term, suggesting instead the term 'roll-off', because 'the late floor-reaction peak is the result of leverage by body alignment, rather than an active downward thrust'. However, it is clear that the 'push off' is not simply passive, since it is the period during which the generation of power at the ankle is greatest

(Winter, 1983). What is not clear is whether this power is used to accelerate the whole body (as suggested by Winter) or merely the leg (as suggested by Perry) or (as seems most likely) some combination of the two. Buczek et al. (2003) showed that power generation at the ankle is necessary to sustain normal walking. Using terms borrowed from the study of posture control, normal walking involves an 'ankle strategy' but may be replaced by a 'hip strategy' in which subjects 'decrease their push-off, pulling their leg forward from their hips' (Mueller et al., 1994).

2. Upper body: The attitude of the upper body at opposite initial contact resembles that described for initial contact, except that the trunk is now moving towards the left rather than the right, and the trunk is twisted so that the right shoulder and arm and the left side of the pelvis are forward.

3. Hip: At opposite initial contact, the hip reaches its most extended position (typically between 10° and 20° of extension, depending on how it is measured) and motion reverses in the direction of flexion (Fig. 2.5). With the hip extended, adductor longus acts as the primary hip flexor (Perry, 1992) and probably generates sufficient moment to initiate hip flexion, particularly when combined with tension in the stretched hip ligaments and the effects of gravity.

4. Knee: The knee is already moving into flexion by the time of opposite initial contact (Fig. 2.5). The force vector has moved behind the knee, aiding its flexion (Fig. 2.16) and rectus femoris begins to contract eccentrically (included with quadriceps in Fig. 2.10), to prevent flexion from occurring too rapidly. The term 'pull off' has been used for the hip and knee flexion occurring during pre-swing.

5. Ankle and foot: From before opposite initial contact until the foot leaves the ground at toe off, the ankle is moving into plantarflexion (Fig. 2.5), due to concentric contraction of the triceps surae (Fig. 2.10). Extension of the toes at the MTP joints continues and causes a tightening of the plantar fascia. The foot reaches its maximal supination, with hindfoot inversion (adduction or varus angulation) and coupled external tibial rotation. These various factors combine to lock the midtarsal joints, resulting in high stability of the foot for loadbearing (Inman et al., 1981; Rose and Gamble, 1994).

6. Moments and powers: A peak of hip internal flexor moment occurs around opposite initial contact (Fig. 2.7). As stated above (p. 45, Opposite initial contact, section 3), it probably results from a

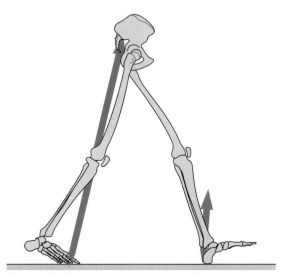

Fig. 2.16 • Opposite initial contact: position of right leg (green), left leg (grey) and ground reaction force vector.

combination of adductor longus contraction, passive tension in the hip ligaments and gravity. As the direction of hip motion reverses from extension to flexion, power absorption (H2 in Fig. 2.8) is replaced by power generation (H3 in Fig. 2.8). During terminal stance, flexion of the knee brings the joint in front of the force vector (Fig. 2.16), reversing the external moment from extensor to flexor and hence changing the internal moment from flexor to extensor (Fig. 2.7). Eccentric contraction of rectus femoris (included with quadriceps in Fig. 2.10) limits the rate of knee flexion and results in power absorption (K3 in Fig. 2.8). At the ankle, the force vector is well in front of the joint at opposite initial contact (Fig. 2.16). The resulting high external dorsiflexor moment is opposed by a correspondingly high internal plantarflexor moment (Fig. 2.7), produced by concentric contraction of the triceps surae (Fig. 2.9). The result is a large generation of power (A2 in Fig. 2.8), which is the highest power generation of the entire gait cycle. The immediate effect of this power generation is to accelerate the limb forward into the swing phase.

Toe off (Fig. 2.17)

1. General: Toe off generally occurs at about 60% of the gait cycle (57% in the subject used for illustration). It separates pre-swing from initial swing and is the point at which the stance phase ends and the

swing phase begins. The name 'terminal contact' has been proposed for this event, since in pathological gait the toe may not be the last part of the foot to leave the ground.

2. Upper body: The extreme rotations of the shoulders, arms and trunk all begin to return towards the neutral position, as the trunk gains height and moves towards the new (left) supporting foot.

3. Hip: As the foot leaves the ground, the hip continues to flex (Fig. 2.5). This is achieved by gravity and tension in the hip ligaments, as well as by contraction of the rectus femoris (included with quadriceps in Fig. 2.10) and adductor longus.

4. Knee: By the time of toe off, the knee has flexed to around half of the angle it will achieve at the peak of swing phase flexion. This flexion is aided by the positioning of the ground reaction force vector well behind the knee (Fig. 2.17), although the magnitude of the force declines rapidly, reaching zero as the foot leaves the ground. The major part of knee flexion then results from hip flexion: the leg acts as a jointed 'double pendulum' so that as the hip flexes, the shank is 'left behind', due to its inertia, resulting in flexion of the knee. At the very beginning of the swing phase, rectus femoris may contract eccentrically to prevent excessive knee flexion, particularly at faster walking speeds (Nene et al., 1999).

5. Ankle and foot: The peak of ankle plantarflexion occurs just after toe off. The magnitude of plantarflexion depends on the method of measurement; it is 25° in Figure 2.5. Triceps surae contraction ceases prior to toe off and tibialis anterior begins to contract (Fig. 2.10), to bring the ankle up into a neutral or dorsiflexed attitude during the swing phase.

6. Moments and powers: Around toe off, the hip still shows an internal flexor moment (Fig. 2.7), resulting from gravity, ligament elasticity, adductor longus and iliopsoas contraction. Since the hip is flexing at this time, power generation occurs (H3 in Fig. 2.8). As stated above (p. 46, Toe off, section 4), during pre-swing and initial swing, hip flexion causes the knee to flex, the 'double pendulum' resulting in an external flexor moment at the knee, opposed by an internal extensor moment (Fig. 2.7), as rectus femoris contracts eccentrically (included with quadriceps in Fig. 2.10) to limit the speed at which the knee flexes. This eccentric contraction absorbs power (K3 in Fig. 2.8). At the ankle, the internal plantarflexor moment reduces rapidly during pre-swing as the magnitude of the ground reaction

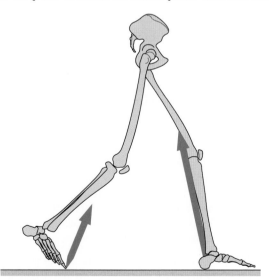

Fig. 2.17 • Toe off: position of right leg (green), left leg (grey) and ground reaction force vector.

force declines, falling to zero as the foot leaves the ground at toe off (Fig. 2.7). The ankle power generation peak also declines to around zero during this period (Fig. 2.8).

Feet adjacent (Fig. 2.18)

1. General: Feet adjacent separates initial swing from mid-swing. It is the time when the swinging leg passes the stance phase leg and the two feet are side by side. The swing phase occupies about 40% of the gait cycle and the feet become adjacent around the centre of this time; in the subject used for illustration, it occurred at 77% of the gait cycle. Alternative names for feet adjacent are 'foot clearance' and 'mid-swing'; the latter term is now applied to a period of the gait cycle, rather than to a particular event. Initial swing is also known as 'lift off'.

2. Upper body: When the feet are adjacent, the trunk is at its highest position and is maximally displaced over the stance phase leg (left). The arms are level with each other, one (left) moving forward and one (right) moving back.

3. Hip: The hip starts to flex even prior to toe off and by the time the feet are adjacent, it is well flexed (20° in Fig. 2.5). This is achieved by a powerful contraction of iliopsoas (Fig. 2.10), aided by gravity.

4. Knee: The flexion of the knee during the swing phase results largely from the flexion of the hip. As described above (p. 46, Toe off, section 6), the

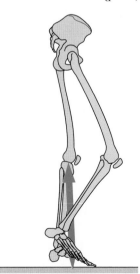

Fig. 2.18 • Feet adjacent: position of right leg (green) and left leg (grey).

leg acts as a jointed pendulum and no muscular contraction is necessary around the knee (thus enabling above-knee amputees to achieve swing phase knee flexion in their prosthetic limb). The peak swing phase knee flexion angle is usually between 60° and 70°. It occurs before the feet are adjacent, by which time the knee has started to extend again. In fast walking, swing phase knee flexion is less than when walking at a natural speed, to shorten the swing phase. This is achieved by co-contraction of the rectus femoris and hamstrings (Gage, 2004).

5. Ankle and foot: At the time the feet are adjacent, the ankle is moving from a plantarflexed attitude around toe off towards a neutral or dorsiflexed attitude in terminal swing. Most of the shortening of the swing phase leg required to achieve toe clearance comes from flexion of the knee, but the ankle also needs to move out of plantarflexion. This movement requires contraction of the anterior tibial muscles, although the force of contraction is much less than that required to control foot lowering following initial contact. The closest approach of the toes to the ground occurs around the time the feet are adjacent. In normal walking, the toes clear the ground by very little; Murray (1967) found a mean clearance of 14 mm with a range of 1–38 mm. The degree of foot supination reduces following toe off, but the foot remains slightly supinated until the following initial contact.

6. Moments and powers: As the hip moves into flexion, from opposite initial contact, through pre-swing and initial swing until the feet are adjacent, an internal flexor moment is present (Fig. 2.7). This is generated by gravity, rectus femoris and the adductors, with the addition of ligament elasticity at the beginning of the movement and iliopsoas contraction towards its end (Fig. 2.9). Hip flexion, in response to this moment, results in the highest peak of power generation at the hip (H3 in Fig. 2.8), the power being used to accelerate the swinging leg forward. The resulting kinetic energy is later transferred to the trunk, as the swinging leg is decelerated again at the end of the swing phase. Between toe off and feet adjacent, the knee continues to show a small internal extensor moment, as rectus femoris (part of quadriceps in Fig. 2.10) prevents the knee from flexing too rapidly in response to the external flexor moment transferred from the hip (see above). While the knee is still flexing, power absorption occurs (K3 in Fig. 2.8). Only very small moments and power exchanges are seen at the ankle, since only the weight of the foot is involved.

Tibia vertical (Fig. 2.19)

1. General: The division between the periods of mid-swing and terminal swing is marked by the tibia of the swinging leg becoming vertical, which occurred at 86% of the gait cycle in the subject used for illustration. Terminal swing is also known as 'reach'.

2. Upper body: When the tibia is vertical on the swing phase leg (right), the trunk has begun to lose vertical height and to move from its maximum displacement over the supporting (left) leg back towards the midline. The left arm is now in front of the right and the right side of the pelvis is a little in front of the left side (Fig. 2.19).

3. Hip: Tibia vertical marks approximately the time at which further hip flexion ceases, the subject used for illustration having a hip angle of about 27° of flexion from tibia vertical to the next initial contact (Fig. 2.5). The hamstrings contract increasingly strongly during terminal swing (Fig. 2.10) to limit the rate of knee extension, while maintaining the hip joint in this flexed position.

4. Knee: Tibia vertical occurs during a period of rapid knee extension, as the knee goes from the peak of swing phase flexion, prior to feet adjacent, to more or less full extension prior to the next initial contact (Fig. 2.5). This extension is largely passive, being the return swing of the lower (shank) segment of the double pendulum referred to above (p. 46,

Toe off, section 4). Eccentric contraction of the hamstrings prevents this motion from causing an abrupt hyperextension of the knee at the end of swing (Fig. 2.10).

5. Ankle and foot: Once toe clearance has occurred, generally before the tibia becomes vertical, the ankle attitude becomes less important: it may be anywhere between a few degrees of plantarflexion and a few degrees of dorsiflexion, prior to the next initial contact (Fig. 2.5). Tibialis anterior continues to contract, to hold the ankle in position, but its activity usually increases prior to initial contact, in anticipation of the greater contraction forces which will be needed during the loading response (Fig. 2.10).

6. Moments and powers: At the hip, by the time of tibia vertical, an increasing internal extensor moment is seen (Fig. 2.7), largely generated by contraction of the hamstrings, although gluteus maximus also begins to contract prior to the next initial contact (Fig. 2.10). This moment probably permits the transfer of momentum from the swinging leg to the trunk, recovering some of the kinetic energy imparted to the leg in initial swing (H3 in Fig. 2.8). Since the hip angle is essentially static during terminal swing, very little power exchange occurs at the joint itself. The knee demonstrates an increasing internal flexor moment (Fig. 2.7), which is generated by eccentric contraction of the hamstrings (Fig. 2.10), with power absorption (K4 in Fig. 2.8). This occurs in response to an external extensor moment, generated by the inertia of the swinging shank, which would hyperextend the knee if it were not checked. The ankle moment remains negligible (Fig. 2.7), with very little power exchange (Fig. 2.8).

Terminal foot contact (Fig. 2.11)

The gait cycle ends at the next initial contact of the same foot (in this case, the right foot). Because it is confusing to refer to the *end* of the cycle as '*initial contact*', it is sometimes known as 'terminal foot contact'.

Ground reaction forces

The *force platform* (or forceplate) is an instrument commonly used in gait analysis. It gives the total force applied by the foot to the ground, although it does not show the distribution of different parts of this force (e.g. heel and forefoot) on the walking surface.

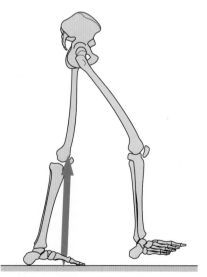

Fig. 2.19 • Tibia vertical: position of right leg (green) and left leg (grey).

Some force platforms give only one component of the force (usually vertical), but most give a full three-dimensional description of the ground reaction force vector. The electrical output signals may be processed to produce three components of force (vertical or 'Fz', medial-lateral or 'Fy', and fore-aft (anterior-posterior), or 'Fx'). As forceplates can be mounted in multiple directions, it is best to describe the forces as F_v, F_{A-P}, and F_{M-L} to avoid confusion. The forceplate also produces the two coordinates of the centre of pressure, and the moments about the vertical axis. The *centre of pressure* is the point on the ground through which a single resultant force appears to act, although in reality the total force is made up of innumerable small force vectors, spread out across a finite area on the surface of the platform.

Since the ground reaction force is a three-dimensional vector, it would be preferable to display it as such for the purposes of interpretation. Unfortunately, this is seldom practical. The most common form of display is that shown in Figure 2.20, where the three components of force are plotted against time for the walk shown in the previous figures. The sign convention used in Figure 2.20 is the same as that used by Winter (1991), where the ground reaction force is positive upwards, forwards and to the right. Regrettably there is no general agreement on sign conventions.

The vertical force shows a characteristic double hump, which results from an upward acceleration of the centre of gravity during early stance (F1), a reduction in downward force as the body 'flies' over the leg in mid-stance (F2) and a second peak due to deceleration (F3), as the downward motion is checked in late stance. The fore-aft (or anteroposterior) trace from the right foot shows 'braking' during the first half of the stance phase (F4) and 'propulsion' during the second half (F5). The left foot shows the same pattern, but with the direction of the lateral force reversed. The lateral component of force is generally very small; for most of the stance phase of the right foot, the ground reaction force accelerates the centre of gravity towards the left side of the body, and during the stance phase of the left foot, the acceleration is towards the right side of the body.

Plots of this type are difficult to interpret and encourage consideration of the force vector as separate components, rather than as a three-dimensional whole. The 'butterfly diagram' shown in Figure 2.9 is an improvement on this, since it combines two of the force components (vertical and fore-aft) with

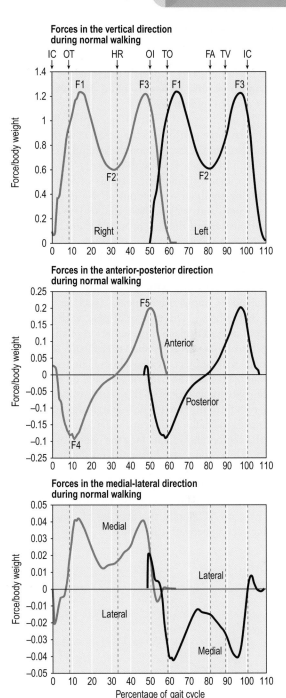

Fig. 2.20 • Vertical, anterior-posterior and medial-lateral components of the ground reaction force, in newtons\body weight, for right foot (green line) and left foot (black line). Abbreviations as in Figure 2.5. See text for sign conventions.

the centre of pressure in the fore-aft direction. It also preserves information on timing, since the lines representing the force vector are at regular intervals (10 ms in this case). Butterfly diagrams for the frontal and transverse planes are more difficult to interpret and are seldom used.

The other type of information commonly derived from the force platform is the position of the centre of pressure of the two feet on the ground, as shown in Figure 2.21, again for the same walk. This may be used to identify abnormal patterns of foot contact, including an abnormal toe out or toe in angle. The step length and walking base can also be measured from this type of display, provided there is an identifiable initial contact.

Should the pattern of foot contact be of particular interest, it is preferable to combine the data on the centre of pressure with an outline of the foot, obtained by some other means (such as chalk or ink on the floor). This type of display, with the addition of a sagittal plane representation of the ground reaction force vector, is shown in Figure 2.22 for a normal male subject wearing shoes. The trace shows initial contact at the back of the heel on the lateral side, with progression of the centre of force along the middle of the foot to the metatarsal heads, where it moves medially, ending at the hallux. The spacing of the vectors shows how long the centre of pressure spends in any one area. It is worth noting that there is a cluster of vectors just in front of the edge of the heel, where the shoe is not in contact with the ground, again pointing out the fact that the centre of pressure is merely the average of a number of forces acting beneath the foot.

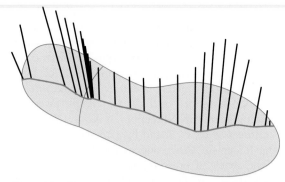

Fig. 2.22 • Foot outline, centre of pressure and sagittal plane representation of ground reaction force vector; right foot of a normal male subject walking in shoes.

There is considerable variation between individuals as to how much force is applied to the ground at initial contact, in some cases this leads to what is known as a heelstrike transient. This is caused by the swinging limb hitting the ground with a backwards velocity, causing a rapid impact peak as the leg decelerates. Figure 2.23 shows the vertical component of the ground reaction force from a fast walk, in hard-heeled shoes, by an individual with a marked heelstrike. The data were recorded at 1000 Hz from a Bertec force platform, which has a particularly high-frequency response. It has been suggested that transient forces in the joints, resulting from the

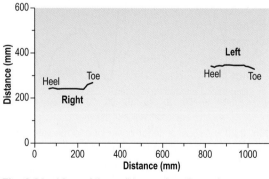

Fig. 2.21 • View of the walking surface from above, showing the centre of pressure beneath the two feet, with the right heel contacting first and the subject walking towards the right of the diagram.

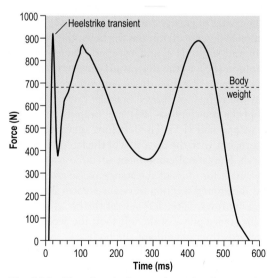

Fig. 2.23 • Plot of vertical ground reaction force against time, showing the heelstrike transient in a particularly 'vigorous' walker wearing hard-heeled shoes. Unfiltered data from Bertec force platform, sampled at 1000 Hz.

heelstrike, may cause degenerative arthritis (Radin, 1987). The heelstrike transient represents the transfer of momentum from the moving leg to the ground. It is a fairly short event, typically lasting 10–20 ms, and can only be observed using measuring equipment with a fast enough response time. A review article on the heelstrike transient and related topics was published by Whittle (1999).

Moments about the vertical axis are seldom reported. In comparing these moments between normal children with children with clubfeet, Sawatzky et al. (1994) were surprised to find only small, and not statistically significant, differences. However, as will be explained in Chapter 4, these moments largely result from the acceleration and deceleration of the swing phase leg and only minor changes could be expected to be introduced by the foot on the ground.

Support moment

Winter (1980) coined the term 'support moment' to describe the sum of the sagittal plane moments about the hip, knee and ankle joints:

$$MS = MH + MK + MA \qquad \text{(Winter)}$$

where MS, MH, MK and MA are the support, hip, knee and ankle moments, respectively.

Winter noted that the support moment was far less variable than its individual components, suggesting that a decreased moment about one joint could be compensated for by an increased moment about one or both of the other joints. However, it was difficult to interpret this in biomechanical terms, since the sign convention was based on flexion and extension, rather than on clockwise and anticlockwise moments, which caused the direction of the knee moment to be opposite to that of the hip and ankle moments. Hof (2000) published a justification for the support moment and suggested that it is responsible for preventing collapse of the knee. Based on his analysis, he suggested the following revised formula for its calculation:

$$MS = \tfrac{1}{2}MH + MK + \tfrac{1}{2}MA \qquad \text{(Hof)}$$

Figure 2.24 illustrates the support moment calculated from the sagittal plane hip, knee and ankle internal moments from the normal subject used for illustration throughout this chapter, using the formula suggested by Hof (2000).

Anderson and Pandy (2003) suggested that a better alternative to the support moment would be the

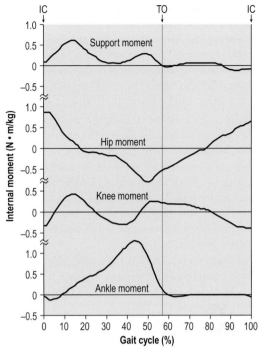

Fig. 2.24 • Support moment, calculated using the formula of Hof (2000), from the sagittal plane internal joint moments of right hip, knee and ankle. Abbreviations and sign conventions as in Figure 2.5.

sum of the vertical components of force from individual muscles during walking.

Energy consumption

It is relatively easy to measure the energy consumption of a vehicle, but much more difficult to make equivalent measurements of human walking, for two reasons. Firstly, there is a clear relationship between the fuel level in the tank of a vehicle and how much energy has been used, whereas knowing how much food a person has eaten gives no information on the energy consumed in a particular activity. Secondly, a vehicle which is switched off uses no energy, whereas people use metabolic energy all the time, whether they are walking or not.

The first problem, that of measuring the 'fuel consumption', can be solved by measuring not the fuel consumed but the oxygen which is used to oxidise it. Measurements of oxygen uptake, while not particularly pleasant for the subject (who has to wear a face mask or mouthpiece), are nonetheless perfectly practical and are used routinely to measure the metabolic cost of different activities.

The second problem, the lack of a suitable baseline for energy consumption measurements in humans, is not easy to solve and requires a different way of thinking about the topic. The energy used by a person who is walking can be divided into three parts.

1. The muscles used for walking consume energy, as they accelerate and decelerate the trunk and the limb segments in different directions.
2. There is an 'overhead' involved in walking, in that the expenditure of energy by the muscles involves increased activity by the heart and the muscles used in breathing, which themselves use energy. Energy is also expended in maintaining the upright posture.
3. The 'basal metabolism' is the irreducible minimum energy a person will consume if they are totally at rest. Basal metabolic rate (BMR) is the energy expended by the body at rest to maintain normal body functions. This continual work makes up about 60–70% of the calories we use and includes respiration, cardiovascular function, and the maintenance of body temperature.

The relationship between metabolic energy and physical energy is very complicated. As explained in Chapter 1 (p. 27), if a muscle undergoes an isometric contraction, it still uses energy, although its length does not change and the physical work it does is zero. In an eccentric contraction, when it lengthens under tension, it uses up metabolic energy, when in physical terms one would expect it to gain energy, rather than to lose it.

In the past it has been usual to estimate the mechanical efficiency of walking by looking at the difference in oxygen consumption between the 'basal' state and walking at a given speed. This approach neglects the various overheads, however, and makes slow walking appear to be extremely inefficient. Inman et al. (1981) and Rose and Gamble (1994) suggested that it is more realistic to use standing or very slow walking as the baseline for measurements of faster walking. Despite these uncertainties, a figure of 25% is often quoted for the efficiency of the conversion of metabolic energy into mechanical energy in a wide range of activities, including walking. A comprehensive review of the energy expenditure of normal and pathological gait was given by Waters and Mulroy (1999).

The energy requirements of walking can be expressed in two ways: the energy used per unit time and the energy used per unit distance. Since energy expenditure is usually inferred from the oxygen used, these are generally known as 'oxygen consumption' and 'oxygen cost', respectively.

Energy consumption per unit time (oxygen consumption)

Inman et al. (1981) and Rose and Gamble (1994) quoted an equation, based on a number of studies, for the relationship between the walking speed and the energy consumption per unit time. The energy consumption included both the basal metabolism and the 'overheads'. They showed, not surprisingly, that energy consumption per unit time is less for slow walking than for fast walking. Translating their equation into SI units, it becomes:

$$E_w = 2.23 + 1.26 \, v^2$$

where E_w is the energy consumption in watts per kilogram body mass and v is the speed in m/s.

As an example of the application of this equation, a 70 kg person walking at 1.4 m/s, which is a typical speed for adults, would consume energy at a rate of 330 w. The term v^2 in the equation shows that energy consumption increases as the square of the walking speed.

Energy consumption per unit distance (oxygen cost)

The energy consumption per metre walked, also known as 'energy cost', has a less straightforward relationship with walking speed, as both very slow and very fast walking speeds use more energy per metre than walking at intermediate speeds. The equation describing this relationship, again converted into SI units, is:

$$E_m = 2.23/v + 1.26 \, v$$

where E_m is the energy consumption in joules per metre per kilogram body mass and v is the speed in m/s. The energy cost of walking is higher in children and decreases steadily with age up to adulthood.

The minimum energy usage is predicted by this equation at a speed of 1.33 m/s. A 70 kg person walking at this speed would use 235 J/m, or 235 kJ/km. A typical 'candy' bar contains around 1000 kJ and would thus supply enough energy to walk 4.26 km, or more than two and a half miles!

The equations quoted above merely give average values for adults, which may be modified by age, sex, walking surface, footwear and so on. Pathological gait is frequently associated with an energy consumption considerably above these 'average' values, due to some combination of abnormal movements, muscle spasticity and co-contraction of antagonistic muscles. To provide a baseline for studies of pathological gait, Waters et al. (1988) made a detailed study of the energy consumption of a total of 260 normal children and adults of both sexes, walking at a variety of speeds.

Optimisation of energy usage

If people were fitted with wheels, very little energy would be needed for locomotion on a level surface and some of the energy expended in going uphill would be recovered when coming down again. For this reason, both wheelchairs and bicycles are remarkably efficient forms of transport, although obviously much less versatile than a pair of legs. During walking, each leg in turn has to be started and stopped and the centre of gravity of the body rises and falls and moves from side to side, all of which use energy. Despite this, walking is not as inefficient as it might be, due to two forms of optimisation: those involving transfers of energy and those which minimise the displacement of the centre of gravity.

Energy transfers

Two types of energy transfer occur during walking: an exchange between potential and kinetic energy and the transfer of energy between one limb segment and another. The most obvious exchange between potential and kinetic energy is in the movement of the trunk. During the double support phase, the trunk is at its lowest vertical position, with its highest forward speed. During the first half of the single support phase, the trunk is lifted up by the supporting leg, converting some of its kinetic energy into potential energy, as its speed reduces. During the latter part of the single support phase, the trunk drops down again in front of the supporting leg and reduces its height while picking up speed again. These exchanges between potential and kinetic energy are the same as in a child's swing, in which the potential energy at the highest point in its travel is converted into kinetic energy as it swings downwards, then back into potential energy again as it swings up the other side.

As well as the vertical motion of the trunk, there are other exchanges between potential and kinetic energy in walking. The twisting of the shoulder girdle and pelvis in opposite directions stores potential energy as tension in the elastic structures, which is converted to kinetic energy as the trunk untwists and then back to potential energy again as the trunk twists the other way.

Winter et al. (1976) studied the energy levels of the limb segments and of the quaintly named HAT (Head, Arms and Trunk). These authors criticised some earlier studies that had included the kinetic energy of linear motion but had neglected the kinetic energy due to rotation, which is responsible for about 10% of the total energy of the shank. Winter et al. studied only the sagittal plane, regarding energy exchanges in the other planes as negligible. They confirmed the exchange between potential and kinetic energy, described above, and estimated that roughly half of the energy of the HAT segment was conserved in this way. The thigh conserved about a third of its energy by exchanges of this sort and the shank virtually none. They also noted that the changes in total body energy were less than the changes in energy of the individual segments, indicating a transfer of energy from one segment to another. In one subject, during a single gait cycle, the energy changes were: shank 16 J, thigh 6 J and HAT 10 J, making a total of 32 J. However, the total body energy change was only 22 J, indicating a saving of 10 J by intersegment transfers. Siegel et al. (2004) performed a detailed analysis on the relationship between lower limb joint moments and mechanical energy during gait.

The six determinants of gait

The six optimisations used to minimise the excursions of the centre of gravity were called the 'determinants of gait' by Saunders et al. (1953) in a classic paper, the main points of which were reiterated, with slight changes, by Inman et al. (1981) and Rose and Gamble (1994). A brief description is given below, but one of these sources should be consulted for a detailed and well-illustrated account. The fourth and fifth determinants were combined in the original descriptions but for the purposes of clarity, the present author has separated them and made other minor changes.

For more than 40 years after their first publication, the determinants of gait were generally accepted and have been redescribed in numerous publications, including previous editions of the present book. However, it has more recently been suggested, in a series of publications (e.g. Della Croce et al., 2001; Gard and Childress, 1997), that although these motions certainly occur, some of them may play little or no part in reducing energy expenditure. Kerrigan (2003) suggested that only the fifth determinant of gait (foot mechanism) significantly reduces the vertical excursions of the centre of mass. Baker et al. (2004) rejected the notion that energy is conserved by restricting the vertical movements of the centre of gravity and proposed instead that energy is mainly conserved by a backwards-and-forwards exchange between potential energy and kinetic energy, as described above. However, having provided these warnings, I will nonetheless reiterate the original descriptions by Saunders et al. (1953)!

The six 'determinants of gait' are as follows.

1. Pelvic rotation

If the knee is kept straight, a movement of the hip from a flexed position to an extended one, such as occurs in the stance phase of gait, will result in the centre of mass of the body moving forwards, but also in its rising and then falling again. The amount of forward movement and the amount of rising and falling both depend on the total angle through which the hip joint moves from flexion to extension (Fig. 2.25A). Since the forward movement is equal to the stride length, it follows that the greater the stride length, the greater will be the angles of flexion and extension of the hip, and the more the centre of mass, will move vertically between its highest and lowest positions. The first 'determinant of gait' is the way in which the pelvis twists about a vertical axis during the gait cycle, bringing each hip joint forwards as that hip flexes and backwards as it extends. This means that for a given stride length, the hip joint itself moves forward through a smaller distance than the foot, so that less flexion and extension of the hip is required. A proportion of the stride length thus comes from the forward-and-backward movement of the hip joint. The reduction in the range of hip flexion and extension leads to a reduction in the vertical movement of the hip (Fig. 2.25B).

2. Pelvic obliquity

As described above, flexion and extension of the hip are accompanied by a rise and fall in the height of the hip joint. If the pelvis were to keep level, the trunk would follow this up-and-down movement. However, the second 'determinant of gait' is the way in which the pelvis tips about an anteroposterior axis, raising first one side and then the other, so that when the hip of the stance phase leg is at its highest point, the pelvis slopes downwards, so that the hip of the swing phase leg is lower than that of the stance phase leg. Since the height of the trunk does not depend on the height of either hip joint alone but on the average of the two of them, this pelvic obliquity reduces the total vertical excursion of the trunk (Fig. 2.26). However, it can only be achieved if the swing phase leg can be shortened sufficiently to clear the ground (normally by both flexing the knee and dorsiflexing the ankle), when the height of its hip joint is reduced.

3. Knee flexion in stance phase

The third, fourth and fifth determinants of gait (Fig. 2.27) are all concerned with adjusting the effective length of the leg, by lengthening it at the beginning and end of the stance phase and shortening it in the middle, to keep the hip height as constant as possible. The third 'determinant' is the stance phase flexion of the knee. As the femur passes from flexion of the hip into extension, if the leg remained straight, the hip joint would rise and then fall, as described above. However, flexion of the knee shortens the leg in the middle of this movement, reducing the height of the apex of the curve.

4. Ankle mechanism

Complementary to the way in which the apex of the curve is lowered by shortening the leg in the middle of the movement from hip flexion to extension, the beginning of the curve is elevated by lengthening the leg at the start of the stance phase – initial contact. This is achieved by the fourth 'determinant of gait' – the ankle mechanism. Because the heel sticks out behind the ankle joint, it effectively lengthens the leg during the loading response (Fig. 2.27).

5. Foot mechanism

In the same way that the heel lengthens the leg at the start of the stance phase, the forefoot lengthens it at the end of stance, in the fifth 'determinant' – the terminal rocker (Fig. 2.27). From the time of heel rise, the effective length of the lower leg increases as the ankle moves from dorsiflexion into plantarflexion.

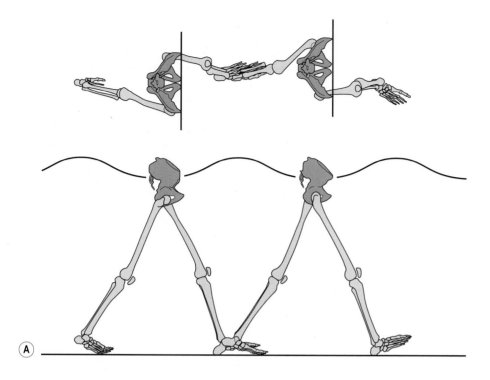

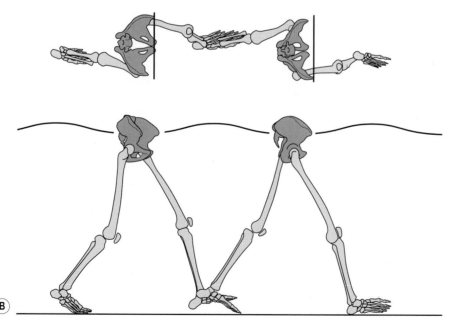

Fig. 2.25 • The first determinant of gait: Pelvic rotation and vertical movement of the centre of mass. If the pelvis did not rotate, the whole of the stride length would come from hip flexion and extension (A). Pelvic rotation about a vertical axis or transverse plane reduces the angle of hip flexion and extension, which in turn reduces the vertical movement of the hip (B).

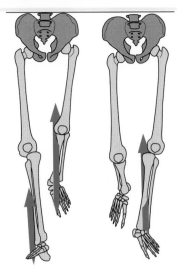

Double support   Single support

Fig. 2.26 • Second determinant of gait: the vertical movement of the trunk is less than that of the hip, due to pelvic obliquity in the coronal plane, about an anteroposterior axis.

6. Lateral displacement of body

The first five determinants of gait are all concerned with reducing the vertical excursions of the centre of gravity. The sixth is concerned with side-to-side movement. If the feet were as far apart as the hips, the body would need to tip from side to side to maintain balance during walking (Fig. 2.28A). By keeping the walking base narrow, little lateral movement is

needed to preserve balance (Fig. 2.28B). The reduction in lateral acceleration and deceleration leads to a reduction in the use of muscular energy. The main adaptation which allows the walking base to be narrow is a slight valgus angulation of the knee, which permits the tibia to be vertical while the femur inclines inwards, from a slightly adducted hip.

It should be obvious that although the six determinants of gait have been described separately, they are all integrated together during each gait cycle. The combined effect is a much smoother trajectory for the centre of gravity and (according to the original description) a much lower energy expenditure. According to Perry (1992), the determinants of gait reduce the vertical excursions of the trunk by about 50% and the horizontal excursions by about 40%.

Starting and stopping

To this point, only steady-state continuous walking has been considered. In order to achieve that state, the individual has to start off, and when they reach their destination, they have to stop. Winter (1995), in a review of balance and posture control, gave a good description of gait initiation and gait termination.

In gait initiation, from standing on both feet, the body weight is shifted to one foot, thus permitting the other foot to be lifted off the ground and moved forward. As an example, suppose the left foot was going to move forwards first (swing limb), while

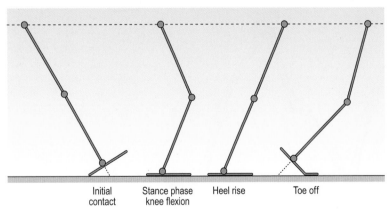

Initial   Stance phase   Heel rise   Toe off
contact   knee flexion

Fig. 2.27 • Third, fourth and fifth determinants of gait: stance phase knee flexion shortens the leg in mid-stance (third determinant); backward projection of the heel at initial contact lengthens the leg (fourth determinant); so does forward projection of the forefoot during pre-swing (fifth determinant).

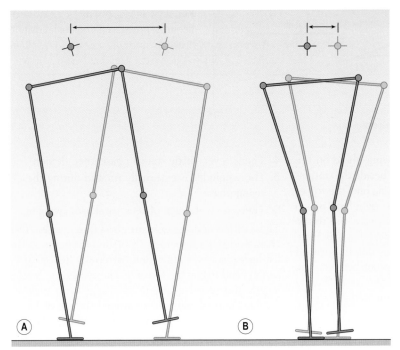

Fig. 2.28 • Sixth determinant of gait: if the feet are placed on the ground far apart (A), large side-to-side movements of the centre of gravity would be necessary to maintain balance; having them closer together (B) reduces the size of these movements.

the body weight is supported by the right foot (stance limb). The shifting of weight over the right foot is achieved by a brief initial push, backwards and to the left, by the left foot. This (following Newton's second law) moves the centre of gravity of the body forwards and to the right. Once the centre of gravity is over the right foot, it is safe to lift the left foot off the ground and move it forward. At the same time, the trunk has started to move forward. The left foot lands on the ground in front of the subject, with a step that is almost exactly the same as in steady-state gait. Body weight is transferred to the left leg, the right foot leaves the ground with a normal toe off, and the subject is walking. By the time the left foot has contacted the ground, the trunk is moving forward at around 85% of the final walking speed and only one or two more steps are needed before the steady-state speed and pattern are achieved. Probably the slowest adjustment is that of side-to-side balance, which may need several steps to stabilise.

One way gait initiation has been assessed is by considering the mechanical process by which the body's centre of mass decouples, or separates, from the

centre of pressure, causing the body to fall forward about the ankle joint (Halliday et al., 1998; Henriksson and Hirschfeld, 2005; Martin et al., 2002; Viton et al., 2000). The process of gait initiation has been generally accepted to consist of two phases, the first of these being the preparatory (postural) phase and second being a stepping (monopodal) phase (Fiolkowski et al., 2002; Mickelborough et al., 2004; Viton et al., 2000). The preparatory phase is when the body begins the decoupling process shifting the centre of pressure initially in the direction of the swinging limb then in the direction of the stance limb (Halliday et al., 1998). The stepping phase is from the point at which the swinging limb is no longer in contact with the floor until its first initial contact (Fig. 2.29). A pathology which causes particular problems for the initiation of gait is parkinsonism; gait initiation in this condition was reviewed by Halliday et al. (1998). Parkinsonian gait will be discussed further in Chapter 6.

Less research has been done on gait termination, although it appears to present a greater challenge to the neural control system. Gait termination involves a stance phase on one side, which is not followed by

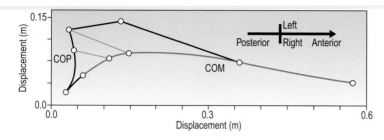

Fig. 2.29 • Centre of mass (COM) and centre of pressure (COP) during gait initiation.

a swing phase, and a shortened swing phase on the other, the moving foot being placed beside the stationary one. If the left foot is the swinging one, the forces to terminate gait are provided by the right foot, which directs the ground reaction force forward and to the right, thus applying a backwards and leftwards force to the body's centre of gravity, arresting its forward motion and bringing it to the midpoint between the feet. The left foot is then planted on the ground beside the right one and the walk has terminated.

Other varieties of gait

As well as normal walking, humans walk backwards, skip, run, ascend and descend slopes and stairs, step over obstacles and carry loads in their hands, on their backs or on their heads. Running has an extensive literature of its own, since it is such an important part of sports medicine. The other types of locomotion have all been studied to a greater or lesser extent, particularly because patients with abnormal neuromuscular systems frequently have greater problems with some of these other activities than they do with normal walking. However, such considerations are beyond the scope of the present introductory text.

Changes in gait with age

Gait in the young

Although a number of studies have been made of the development of gait in children, that by Sutherland et al. (1988) is one of the most detailed. The main ways in which the gait of small children differs from that of adults are as follows:

1. The walking base is wider
2. The stride length and speed are lower and the cycle time shorter (higher cadence)
3. Small children have no heelstrike, initial contact being made by the flat foot

4. There is very little stance phase knee flexion
5. The whole leg is externally rotated during the swing phase
6. There is an absence of reciprocal arm swinging.

These differences in gait mature at different rates. The characteristics numbered (3), (4) and (5) in the above list have changed to the adult pattern by the age of 2, and (1) and (6) by the age of 4. The cycle time, stride length and speed continue to change with growth, reaching normal adult values around the age of 15.

Most children commence walking within 3 months of their first birthday. Prior to this, even tiny babies will make reciprocal stepping motions, if they are moved slowly forwards while held in the standing position with their feet on the ground. However, this is not true walking, as there is little attempt to take any weight on the legs.

Figure 2.30, which is based on data from Sutherland et al. (1988), shows the average sagittal plane motion at the hip, knee and ankle joints in 49 children between 11 and 13 months. It should be compared with Figure 2.5, which shows the same parameters for a normal adult female. Sutherland et al. only gave the timing of initial contact and toe off on the two sides and used a different definition of hip angle; the data in Figure 2.30 have been adjusted into extension by 15° to make them comparable with the other figures in this book.

The pattern of hip flexion and extension differs from that in adults in that the degree of extension is reduced and the hip does not remain flexed for so long at the end of the swing phase. The knee never fully extends, but this is seen at all ages in Sutherland's data and may reflect the method of measurement. There is some stance phase knee flexion in infants, but it is both smaller in magnitude and earlier than in adults. The flexion of the knee in the swing phase is also somewhat reduced at the age of 1 (and most adults have more swing phase flexion than is seen in Fig. 2.5).

Initial contact in small children is by the whole foot, heelstrike being replaced by foot flat. The ankle

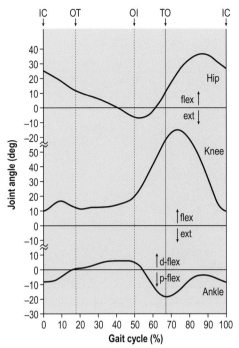

Fig. 2.30 • Sagittal plane hip, knee and ankle angles in 1-year-old children. The hip angle has been moved into extension by 15° to allow for a difference in measurement methods. Sign conventions and abbreviations as in Figure 2.5 (based on data from Sutherland et al., 1988).

is plantarflexed at initial contact and remains so into the early stance phase, in contrast to the adult pattern, in which the ankle is approximately neutral at initial contact but moves rapidly into plantarflexion. The pattern of dorsiflexion followed by plantarflexion through the remainder of the stance phase is essentially the same at all ages.

Since children are smaller than adults, it is not surprising that they walk with a shorter stride length and at a slower speed. Sutherland et al. (1988) showed that stride length is closely related to height and that the ratio of stride length to stature is similar to that found in adults. The change in stride length with age mirrors the change in height, showing a rapid increase up to age 4 and a slower increase thereafter. Todd et al. (1989) detailed the relationships between the height of children and their general gait parameters. Small children walk with a short cycle time (rapid cadence), the mean at the age of one being about 0.70 s (171 steps/min). Cycle time increases with age but is still around 0.85 s (141 steps/min) at age 7, which is well below the typical adult values of 1.06 s (113 steps/min) for men and 1.02 s

(118 steps/min) for women. The shorter cycle time partly compensates for the short stride length and the speed ranged from 0.64 m/s at age 1 to 1.14 m/s at age 7, compared with the typical adult values of 1.46 m/s for males and 1.30 m/s for females. Sutherland did not report on the gait of children beyond the age of 7 and did not distinguish between the results from boys and girls. Table 1 gives the normal ranges for the general gait parameters in children, derived in part from Sutherland's data. However, values based on age alone may be misleading; stride length depends on both height and walking speed, both of which may be lower in children with a disability than in normal children of the same age.

As can be seen in Figure 2.30, the swing phase occupies a smaller proportion of the gait cycle in very small children than in adults, thus minimising the time spent in the less stable condition of single legged stance. The relative duration of the swing phase increases with age, reaching the adult proportion around the age of 4 years. There is symmetry between the two sides at all ages. Sutherland et al. (1988) related the width of the walking base to the width of the body at the top of the pelvis, using the somewhat confusing 'pelvic-span/ankle-spread' ratio. Changing the measurement units for the sake of clarity, the walking base is about 70% of the pelvic width at the age of 1 year, falling to about 45% by the age of 3½, at which level it remains until the age of 7. An average value for adults is not readily available but it is probably less than 30%.

At the very youngest ages, the EMG patterns showed that there is a tendency to activate most muscles for a higher proportion of the gait cycle than in adults. With the exception of the triceps surae, adult patterns are established for most muscles by the age of 2. Sutherland et al. (1988) found that children could be divided into two groups depending on whether the triceps surae was activated in a prolonged (infant) pattern or the normal (adult) pattern. Below the age of 2, over 60% of the children showed the infant pattern; the proportion dropped to below 30% by the age of 7. The authors speculated that this might relate to delayed myelination of the sensory branches of the peripheral nerves.

An excellent review of the main changes in gait occurring during childhood was given by Sutherland (1997). The gait of very small children (under the age of 2) was examined in detail by Grimshaw et al. (1998). The joint moments and powers of this same group were studied by Hallemans et al. (2005).

Gait in the elderly

Cunha (1988) discussed the gait of elderly people and pointed out that many pathological gait disorders are incorrectly thought to be part of the normal ageing process. Identification of an underlying cause, which may be treatable, could result in an improved life for the patient and a reduced risk of falls and fractures. Cunha classified the causes of the gait disorders of old age as follows: neurological, psychological, orthopaedic, endocrinological, general, drugs, senile gait and associated conditions. He described the features of the gait in many conditions affecting the elderly and suggested a plan for the investigation and management of these patients.

A number of investigations have been made of the changes in gait which occur with advancing age, especially by Murray et al. (1969), who studied the gait of men up to the age of 87. The description which follows is confined to the effects of age on free-speed walking, although Murray et al. also examined fast walking. A companion paper (Murray et al., 1970) studied the gait of women up to age 70. It did not provide as much information on the effects of age, but generally confirmed the observations made on males.

The gait of elderly people is subject to two influences: the effects of age itself and the effects of pathological conditions, such as osteoarthritis and parkinsonism, which become more common with advancing age. Provided patients with pathological conditions are carefully excluded, the gait of elderly people appears to be simply a 'slowed down' version of the gait of younger adults. Murray et al. (1969) were careful to point out that 'the walking performance of older men did not resemble a pathological gait'.

Typically, the onset of age-related changes in gait takes place in the decade from 60 to 70 years of age. There is a decreased stride length, a variable but generally increased cycle time (decreased cadence) and an increase in the walking base. Many other changes can also be observed, such as a relative increase in the duration of the stance phase as a percentage of the gait cycle, but most of them are secondary to the changes in stride length, cycle time and walking base. The speed (stride length divided by cycle time) is almost always reduced in elderly people. Table 1 gives normal ranges for the general gait parameters up to the age of 80.

Some of the differences between the gait of the young and the elderly are apparent in Figure 2.31, which is taken from Murray et al. (1969). These

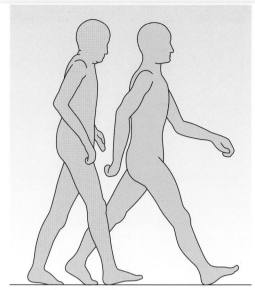

Fig. 2.31 • Body position at right initial contact in older men (left) and younger men (right) (Murray et al., 1969).

authors suggested that the purpose of gait changes in the elderly is to improve the security of walking. Both decreasing the stride length and increasing the walking base make it easier to maintain balance while walking. Increasing the cycle time (reducing the cadence) leads to a reduction in the percentage of the gait cycle for which there is only single limb support, since the increase in cycle length is largely achieved by lengthening the stance phase and hence the double support time.

Changes in the angular excursions of the joints in the elderly include a reduction in the total range of hip flexion and extension, a reduction in swing phase knee flexion and reduced ankle plantarflexion during the push off. However, all of these depend on both cycle time and stride length and are probably within normal limits if these factors are taken into account. Nigg et al. (1994) confirmed these observations in a detailed study on three-dimensional joint ranges of motion in walking, in male and female subjects from 20 to 79 years of age. The vertical movement of the head is reduced and its lateral movement increased, probably secondary to the changes in stride length and walking base, respectively.

The trajectory of the toe over the ground is modified in old age, giving an improved ground clearance during the first half of the swing phase. This is probably another mechanism for improving security. The heel rises less during pre-swing and the foot attitude

Table 1

Normal ranges for gait parameters

Approximate range (95% limits) for general gait parameters in free-speed walking by normal FEMALE subjects of different ages

Age (years)	Cadence (steps/min)	Cycle time (s)	Stride length (m)	Speed (m/s)
13–14	103–150	0.80–1.17	0.99–1.55	0.90–1.62
15–17	100–144	0.83–1.20	1.03–1.57	0.92–1.64
18–49	98–138	0.87–1.22	1.06–1.58	0.94–1.66
50–64	97–137	0.88–1.24	1.04–1.56	0.91–1.63
65–80	96–136	0.88–1.25	0.94–1.46	0.80–1.52

Approximate range (95% limits) for general gait parameters in free-speed walking by normal MALE subjects of different ages

Age (years)	Cadence (steps/min)	Cycle time (s)	Stride length (m)	Speed (m/s)
13–14	100–149	0.81–1.20	1.06–1.64	0.95–1.67
15–17	96–142	0.85–1.25	1.15–1.75	1.03–1.75
18–49	91–135	0.89–1.32	1.25–1.85	1.10–1.82
50–64	82–126	0.95–1.46	1.22–1.82	0.96–1.68
65–80	81–125	0.96–1.48	1.11–1.71	0.81–1.61

Approximate range (95% limits) for general gait parameters in free-speed walking by normal CHILDREN of different ages (ages 1–7 years based on Sutherland et al. (1988))

Age (years)	Cadence (steps/min)	Cycle time (s)	Stride length (m)	Speed (m/s)
1	127–223	0.54–0.94	0.29–0.58	0.32–0.96
1.5	126–212	0.57–0.95	0.33–0.66	0.39–1.03
2	125–201	0.60–0.96	0.37–0.73	0.45–1.09
2.5	124–190	0.63–0.97	0.42–0.81	0.52–1.16
3	123–188	0.64–0.98	0.46–0.89	0.58–1.22
3.5	122–186	0.65–0.98	0.50–0.96	0.65–1.29
4	121–184	0.65–0.99	0.54–1.04	0.67–1.32
5	119–180	0.67–1.01	0.59–1.10	0.71–1.37
6	117–176	0.68–1.03	0.64–1.16	0.75–1.43
7	115–172	0.70–1.04	0.69–1.22	0.80–1.48
8	113–169	0.71–1.06	0.75–1.30	0.82–1.50
9	111–166	0.72–1.08	0.82–1.37	0.83–1.53
10	109–162	0.74–1.10	0.88–1.45	0.85–1.55
11	107–159	0.75–1.12	0.92–1.49	0.86–1.57
12	105–156	0.77–1.14	0.96–1.54	0.88–1.60

is closer to the horizontal at initial contact, both of these changes being related to the reduction in stride length. There is also an increase in the angle of toe out in elderly people and changes in the posture and movements of the arms, the elbows being more flexed and the shoulders more extended. The reasons for these differences are not known.

The dividing line between normal and abnormal may be difficult to define in elderly people. A condition known as 'idiopathic gait disorder of the elderly' has been described, which is essentially an exaggeration of the gait changes which normally occur with age and is characterised by a cautious attitude to walking, with a prolonged cycle time (low cadence), a short stride length and an increased step-to-step variability. For a comprehensive review of the changes in gait with advancing age, see Prince et al. (1997).

References

Anderson, F.C., Pandy, M.G., 2003. Individual muscle contributions to support in normal walking. Gait Posture 17, 159–169.

Baker, R., Kirkwood, C., Pandy, M., 2004. Minimizing the vertical excursion of the center of mass is not the primary aim of walking. In: Eighth International Symposium on the 3-D Analysis of Human Movement. Tampa, Florida, USA, March 31–April 2, pp. 101–104.

Basmajian, J.V., 1985. Muscles Alive: Their Functions Revealed by Electromyography. Lippincott Williams & Wilkins, Baltimore, MD.

Blanc, Y., Balmer, C., Landis, T., Vingerhoets, F., 1999. Temporal parameters and patterns of foot roll over during walking: normative data for healthy adults. Gait Posture 10, 97–108.

Bresler, B., Frankel, J.P., 1950. The forces and moments in the leg during level walking. American Society of Mechanical Engineers Transactions 72, 27–36.

Buczek, F.L., Sanders, J.O., Concha, M.C., et al., 2003. Inadequacy of an inverted pendulum model of human gait. In: Gait and Clinical Movement Analysis Society. Eighth Annual Meeting, Wilmington, Delaware, USA, pp. 185–186.

Burnfield, J.M., Tsai, Y.J., Powers, C.M., 2005. Comparison of utilized coefficient of friction during different walking tasks in persons with and without a disability. Gait Posture 22, 82–88.

Cavagna, G.A., Margaria, R., 1966. Mechanics of walking. J. Appl. Physiol. 21, 271–278.

Cham, R., Redfern, M.S., 2002. Changes in gait when anticipating slippery floors. Gait Posture 15, 159–171.

Cunha, U.V., 1988. Differential diagnosis of gait disorders in the elderly. Geriatrics 43, 33–42.

De Luca, C.J., 1997. The use of surface electromyography in biomechanics. J. Appl. Biomech. 13 (2), 135–163.

Della Croce, U., Riley, P.O., Lelas, J.L., et al., 2001. A refined view of the determinants of gait. Gait Posture 14, 79–84.

Fiolkowski, P., Brunt, D., Bishop, M., Woo, R., 2002. Does postural instability affect the initiation of human gait? Neurosci. Lett. 323 (3), 167–170.

Gage, J.R. (Ed.), 2004. The Treatment of Gait Problems in Cerebral Palsy. MacKeith Press, London.

Gard, S.A., Childress, D.S., 1997. The effect of pelvic list on the vertical displacement of the trunk during normal walking. Gait Posture 5, 233–238.

Garrison, F.H., 1929. An Introduction to the History of Medicine. WB Saunders, Philadelphia, PA.

Grimshaw, P.N., Marques-Bruna, P., Salo, A., et al., 1998. The 3-dimensional kinematics of the walking gait cycle of children aged between 10 and 24 months: cross sectional and repeated measures. Gait Posture 7, 7–15.

Hallemans, A., De Clercq, D., Otten, B., et al., 2005. 3D joint dynamics of walking in toddlers. A cross-sectional study spanning the first rapid development phase of walking. Gait Posture 22, 107–118.

Halliday, S.E., Winter, D.A., Frank, J.S., et al., 1998. The initiation of gait in young, elderly and Parkinson's disease subjects. Gait Posture 8, 8–14.

Henriksson, M., Hirschfeld, H., 2005. Physically active older adults display alterations in gait initiation. Gait Posture 21 (3), 289–296.

Hof, A.L., 2000. On the interpretation of the support moment. Gait Posture 12, 196–199.

Inman, V.T., Ralston, H.J., Todd, F., 1981. Human Walking. Williams & Wilkins, Baltimore, MD.

Kerrigan, C.D., 2003. Discoveries from quantitative gait analysis. Gait Posture 18 (Suppl. 1), S13.

Lamoth, C.J.C., Beek, P.J., Meijer, O.G., 2002. Pelvis-thorax coordination in the transverse plane during gait. Gait Posture 16, 101–114.

Macellari, V., Giacomozzi, C., Saggini, R., 1999. Spatial-temporal parameters of gait: reference data and a statistical method for normality assessment. Gait Posture 10, 171–181.

Martin, M., Shinberg, M., Kuchibhatla, M., Ray, L., Carollo, J.J., Schenkman, M.L., 2002. Gait initiation in community-dwelling adults with Parkinson disease: comparison with older and younger adults without the disease. Phys. Ther. 82 (6), 566–577.

Mickelborough, J., van der Linden, M.L., Tallis, R.C., Ennos, A.R., 2004. Muscle activity during gait initiation in normal elderly people. Gait Posture 19 (1), 50–57.

Mueller, M.J., Sinacore, D.R., Hoogstrate, S., et al., 1994. Hip and ankle walking strategies: effect on peak plantar pressures and implications for neuropathic ulceration. Arch. Phys. Med. Rehabil. 75, 1196–1200.

Murray, M.P., 1967. Gait as a total pattern of movement. Am. J. Phys. Med. 46, 290–333.

Murray, M.P., Kory, R.C., Clarkson, B.H., 1969. Walking patterns in healthy old men. J. Gerontol. 24, 169–178.

Murray, M.P., Kory, R.C., Sepic, S.B., 1970. Walking patterns of normal women. Arch. Phys. Med. Rehabil. 51, 637–650.

Nene, A., Mayagoitia, R., Veltink, P., 1999. Assessment of rectus femoris function during initial swing phase. Gait Posture 9, 1–9.

Nigg, B.M., Fisher, V., Ronsky, J.L., 1994. Gait characteristics as a function of age and gender. Gait Posture 2, 213–220.

Oeffinger, D., Brauch, B., Cranfill, S., et al., 1999. Comparison of gait with and without shoes in children. Gait Posture 9, 95–100.

Paul, J.P., 1965. Bio-engineering studies of the forces transmitted by joints. (II) Engineering analysis. In: Kenedi, J.P. (Ed.), Biomechanics and Related Bioengineering Topics. Pergamon, Oxford, pp. 369–380.

Paul, J.P., 1966. Forces transmitted by joints in the human body. Proceedings of the Institute of Mechanical Engineers 181, 8–15.

Pedotti, A., 1977. Simple equipment used in clinical practice for the evaluation of locomotion. IEEE Transactions on Biomedical Engineering BME-24 456–461.

Perry, J., 1974. Kinesiology of lower extremity bracing. Clin. Orthop. Relat. Res. 102, 18–31.

Perry, J., 1992. Gait Analysis: Normal and Pathological Function. Slack Incorporated, Thorofare, NJ.

Prince, F., Winter, D.A., Stergiou, P., et al., 1994. Anticipatory control of upper body balance during human locomotion. Gait Posture 2, 19–25.

Prince, F., Corriveau, H., Hébert, R., et al., 1997. Gait in the elderly. Gait Posture 5, 128–135.

Radin, E.L., 1987. Osteoarthrosis: what is known about its prevention. Clin. Orthop. Relat. Res. 222, 60–65.

Rose, J., Gamble, J.G., 1994. Human Walking, second ed. Williams & Wilkins, Baltimore, MD.

Rose, Gamble, 2005. Human Walking, third ed. Lippincott Williams and Wilkins.

Sadeghi, H., 2003. Local or global asymmetry in gait of people without impairments. Gait Posture 17, 197–204.

Saunders, J.B.D.M., Inman, V.T., Eberhart, H.S., 1953. The major determinants in normal and pathological gait. J. Bone Joint Surg. Am. 35, 543–558.

Sawatzky, B.J., Sanderson, D.J., Beauchamp, R.D., et al., 1994. Ground reaction forces in gait in children with clubfeet – a preliminary study. Gait Posture 2, 123–127.

Sekiya, N., Nagasaki, H., 1998. Reproducibility of the walking patterns of normal young adults: test-retest reliability of the walk ratio (step-length/step-rate). Gait Posture 7, 225–227.

Shiavi, R., 1985. Electromyographic patterns in adult locomotion: a comprehensive review. J. Rehabil. Res. Dev. 22, 85–98.

Siegel, K.L., Kepple, T.M., Stanhope, S.J., 2004. Joint moment control of mechanical energy flow during normal gait. Gait Posture 19, 69–75.

Steindler, A., 1953. A historical review of the studies and investigations made in relation to human gait. J. Bone Joint Surg. Am. 35, 540–542.

Sutherland, D.H., 1984. Gait Disorders in Childhood and Adolescence. Williams & Wilkins, Baltimore, MD.

Sutherland, D.H., 1997. The development of mature gait. Gait Posture 6, 163–170.

Sutherland, D.H., 2001. The evolution of clinical gait analysis. Part I: Kinesiological EMG. Gait Posture 14, 61–70.

Sutherland, D.H., 2002. The evolution of clinical gait analysis. Part II: Kinematics. Gait Posture 16, 159–1179.

Sutherland, D.H., 2005. The evolution of clinical gait analysis. Part III: Kinetics and energy assessment. Gait Posture 21, 447–461.

Sutherland, D.H., Olshen, R.A., Biden, E.N., et al., 1988. The Development of Mature Walking. MacKeith Press, London.

Todd, F.N., Lamoreux, L.W., Skinner, S.R., et al., 1989. Variations in the gait of normal children. J. Bone Joint Surg. Am. 71, 196–204.

Viton, J.M., Timsit, M., Mesure, S., Massion, J., Franceschi, J.P., Delarque, A., 2000. Asymmetry of gait initiation in patients with unilateral knee arthritis. Arch. Phys. Med. Rehabil. 81 (2), 194–200.

Wall, J.C., Charteris, J., Turnbull, G.I., 1987. Two steps equals one stride equals what? The applicability of normal gait nomenclature to abnormal walking patterns. Clin. Biomech. (Bristol, Avon) 2, 119–125.

Waters, R.L., Mulroy, S., 1999. The energy expenditure of normal and pathological gait. Gait Posture 9, 207–231.

Waters, R.L., Lunsford, B.R., Perry, J., et al., 1988. Energyspeed relationship of walking: standard tables. J. Orthop. Res. 6, 215–222.

Wells, R.P., 1981. The projection of the ground reaction force as a predictor of internal joint moments. Bull. Prosthet. Res. 10–35, 15–19.

Whittle, M.W., 1999. Generation and attenuation of transient impulsive forces beneath the foot: a review. Gait Posture 10, 264–275.

Winter, D.A., 1980. Overall principle of lower limb support during stance phase of gait. J. Biomech. 13, 923–927.

Winter, D.A., 1983. Energy generation and absorption at the ankle and knee during fast, natural and slow cadences. Clin. Orthop. Relat. Res. 175, 147–154.

Winter, D.A., 1991. The Biomechanics and Motor Control of Human Gait, second ed. University of Waterloo Press, Waterloo, Ontario.

Winter, D.A., 1995. Human balance and posture control during standing and walking. Gait Posture 3, 193–214.

Winter, D.A., Quanbury, A.O., Reimer, G.D., 1976. Analysis of instantaneous energy of normal gait. J. Biomech. 9, 253–257.

Pathological and other abnormal gaits

3

Michael Whittle   David Levine   Jim Richards

Although some variability is present in normal gait, particularly in the use of the muscles, there is an identifiable 'normal pattern' of walking and a 'normal range' can be defined for all of the variables which can be measured. Pathology of the locomotor system frequently produces gait patterns which are clearly 'abnormal'. Some of these abnormalities can be identified by eye, but others can only be identified by the use of appropriate measurement systems.

In order for a person to walk, the locomotor system must be able to accomplish four things:

1. Each leg in turn must be able to support the body weight without collapsing
2. Balance must be maintained, either statically or dynamically, during single leg stance
3. The swinging leg must be able to advance to a position where it can take over the supporting role
4. Sufficient power must be provided to make the necessary limb movements and to advance the trunk.

In normal walking, all of these are achieved without any apparent difficulty and with a modest energy consumption. However, in many forms of pathological gait they can be accomplished only by means of abnormal movements, which usually increase the energy consumption, or by the use of walking aids such as canes, crutches or orthoses (calipers and braces). If even one of these four requirements cannot be met, the subject is unable to walk.

The pattern of gait is the outcome of a complex interaction between the many neuromuscular and structural elements of the locomotor system. Abnormal gait may result from a disorder in any part of this system, including the brain, spinal cord, nerves, muscles, joints and skeleton. Abnormal gait may also result from the presence of pain, so that although a person is physically capable of walking normally, they find it more comfortable to walk in some other way.

The term *limp* is commonly used to describe a wide variety of abnormal gait patterns. However, dictionary definitions are unhelpful, a typical one being 'to walk lamely'. Since the word has no clearly defined scientific meaning, it should only be used with caution in the context of gait analysis. The most appropriate use of the word is probably for a gait abnormality involving some degree of asymmetry, which is readily apparent to an untrained observer.

Since gait is the end result of a complicated process, a number of different original problems may manifest themselves in the same abnormality of gait. For this reason, the abnormal gait patterns will be described separately from the pathological conditions which cause them. This chapter describes, in some detail, the most common abnormal gait patterns. This is followed by a description of the use of walking aids such as canes and walkers, and treadmill gait.

Specific gait abnormalities

The following sections are based on a manual of lecture notes for student orthotists published by New York University (1986). Despite being over 25 years old, the manual includes a very useful list of common gait abnormalities, all of which can be identified by eye, which still hold today. The manual criticises the common practice of identifying gait abnormalities by their pathological cause, for example 'hemiplegic gait', which immediately suggests that all hemiplegics walk in the same way, which is far from true, and also neglects the changes in gait which may occur with the passage of time, or result from treatment. The manual suggests that it is preferable to use purely descriptive terms, such as 'excessive medial foot contact'. This practice will be adopted in the following sections. Some of the gait abnormalities described in the New York University publication apply only to the gait of subjects wearing orthoses; these descriptions have been omitted from the present text.

The pathological gait patterns to be described may occur either alone or in combination. If in combination, they may interact, so that the individual gait modifications do not exactly fit the description. The list that follows is not exhaustive; a subject may use a variation of one of the general patterns or may use another gait pattern which is not listed here.

When studying a pathological gait, particularly one which does not appear to fit into one of the standard patterns, it is helpful to remember that an abnormal movement may be performed for one of two reasons:

1. The subject has no choice, the movement being 'forced' on them by weakness, spasticity or deformity
2. The movement is a compensation, which the subject is using to correct for some other problem, which therefore needs to be identified.

Lateral trunk bending

Bending the trunk towards the side of the supporting limb during the stance phase is known as lateral trunk bending, ipsilateral lean or, more commonly, a *Trendelenburg gait*. The purpose of the manoeuvre is generally to reduce the forces in the abductor muscles and hip joint during single leg stance.

Lateral trunk bending is best observed from the front or the back. During the double support phase, the trunk is generally upright but as soon as the swing leg leaves the ground, the trunk leans over towards the side of the stance phase leg, returning to the upright attitude again at the beginning of the next double support phase. The trunk bending may be unilateral, being restricted to the stance phase of one leg, or it may be bilateral, the trunk swaying from one side to the other, to produce a gait pattern known as *waddling*.

In the examples which follow, the weight of the trunk is 452 N, corresponding to a mass of 46 kg, and the weight of the right leg is 147 N, corresponding

to a mass of 15 kg. As explained in Chapter 1 (p. 20), weight is a force, calculated by multiplying an object's mass by the acceleration due to gravity, 9.81 m/s^2.

Figure 3.1 shows a schematic of the trunk, pelvis and hip joints when standing on both legs. The abductor muscles are inactive and the weight of the trunk is divided equally between the two hip joints. Figure 3.2 shows what happens in a normal individual when the right foot is lifted off the ground: the force through the left hip joint increases by a factor of six, from 226 N (23 kgf or 51 lbf) to 1510 N (154 kgf or 339 lbf). This increase in force is made up of three components:

1. The whole of the weight of the trunk is now supported by the left hip joint, instead of being shared between the two hips which produces an anti-clockwise moment

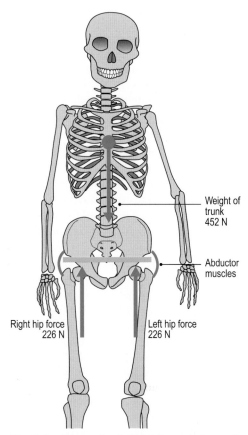

Right hip force 226 N
Weight of trunk 452 N
Abductor muscles
Left hip force 226 N

Fig. 3.1 • Schematic of double legged stance: the force in each hip joint (226 N) is half the weight of the trunk (452 N). The abductors are not contracting.

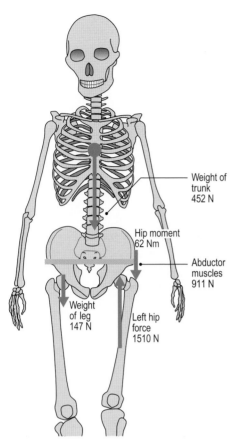

Fig. 3.2 • Schematic of single legged stance on the left (the right leg is held up). The force in the left hip (1510 N) is the sum of: (i) weight of trunk (452 N), (ii) weight of right leg (147 N) and (iii) contraction force of abductor muscles (911 N).

2. The weight of the right leg is now taken by the left hip instead of by the ground, which also produces an anti-clockwise moment
3. The left hip abductors (primarily gluteus medius) contract, produces a clockwise moment to keep the pelvis from dropping on the unsupported side. The reaction force to this contraction passes through the left hip.

These three components contribute to the increased force in the left hip as follows:

1. The force from the trunk increases from 226 N to 452 N (23 kgf or 51 lbf) as this is now not shared
2. Weight of right leg: 147 N (15 kgf or 33 lbf)
3. Contraction of abductors: 911 N (93 kgf or 204 lbf)
4. A total increase of 1284 N (131 kgf or 288 lbf).

It should be noted that this example was invented for the purposes of illustration – the actual numbers should not be taken too seriously!

The four conditions which must be met if this mechanism is to operate satisfactorily are:

- The absence of significant pain on loading
- Adequate power in the hip abductors
- A sufficiently long lever arm for the hip abductors
- A solid and stable fulcrum in or around the hip joint.

Should one or more of these conditions not be met, the subject may adopt lateral trunk bending in an attempt to compensate.

The effect of lateral trunk bending on the joint force is shown in Figure 3.3. There is no effect on

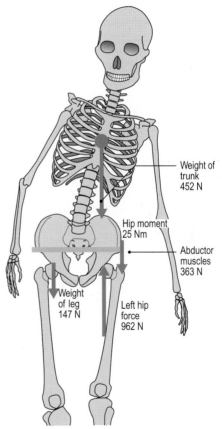

Fig. 3.3 • Lateral trunk bending: bringing the trunk across the supporting hip reduces the anti-clockwise moments about the left hip from 62 Nm to 25 Nm, permitting the pelvis to be stabilised by a smaller abductor force. The force in the left hip (962 N) is the sum of: (i) weight of trunk (452 N), (ii) weight of right leg (147 N), and (iii) contraction force of abductor muscles (363 N).

components (1) and (2) of the increased force, but if the centre of gravity of the trunk is moved directly above the left hip, this eliminates the anti-clockwise moment produced by the mass of the trunk. The abductors are now only required to contract with a force of 363 N (37 kgf or 81 lbf) to balance the anti-clockwise moment provided by the weight of the right leg. There is thus a reduction of 548 N (56 kgf or 123 lbf) in the abductor contraction force and a corresponding reduction in the total joint force, from 1501 N down to 962 N. The numbers in the illustrations refer to standing; during the stance phase of walking, higher forces are to be expected due to the vertical accelerations of the centre of gravity, which cause the force transmitted through the leg to fluctuate above and below body weight (see Fig. 2.19). However, these fluctuations tend to be less in pathological than in normal gait, since the vertical accelerations are less in someone walking with a shorter stride length. The numbers also suppose that the bending of the trunk brings its centre of gravity exactly above the hip joint. This is unlikely to happen in practice, of course, but the principles remain the same, whether the centre of gravity is not deviated as far as the hip joint or even if it passes lateral to it.

There are a number of conditions in which this gait abnormality is adopted.

1. *Painful hip:* If the hip joint is painful, as in osteoarthritis and rheumatoid arthritis, the amount of pain experienced usually depends to a very large extent on the force being transmitted through the joint. Since lateral trunk bending reduces the total joint force, 'Trendelenburg gait' is extremely common in people with arthritis of the hip. Although it produces a useful reduction in force and hence in pain, the forces still remain substantial (962 N in Fig. 3.3) and some form of definitive treatment is usually required.

2. *Hip abductor weakness:* If the hip abductors are weak, they may be unable to contract with sufficient force to stabilise the pelvis during single leg stance. In this case, the pelvis will dip on the side of the foot which is off the ground (Trendelenburg's sign, as opposed to 'Trendelenburg gait'). In order to reduce the demands on the weakened muscles, the subject will usually employ lateral trunk bending, in both standing and walking, to reduce joint moment as far as possible (Fig. 3.4). Hip abductor weakness may be caused by disease or injury affecting either the muscles themselves or the nervous system which controls them.

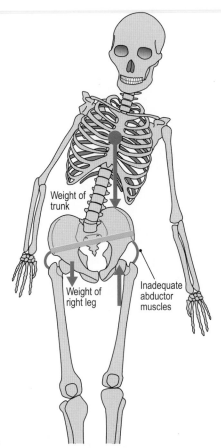

Fig. 3.4 • Trendelenburg's sign: due to inadequate hip abductors, the pelvis drops on the unsupported side when one foot is lifted off the ground. To compensate, the subject bends the trunk over the supporting hip.

3. *Abnormal hip joint:* Three conditions around the hip joint will lead to difficulties in stabilising the pelvis using the abductors: *congenital dislocation of the hip* (CDH, also known as *developmental dysplasia of the hip*), *coxa vara* and *slipped femoral epiphysis*. In all three, the effective length of the gluteus medius is reduced because the greater trochanter of the femur moves proximally, towards the pelvic brim. Since the muscle is shortened, it is unable to function efficiently and thus contracts with a reduced tension. In CDH and severe cases of slipped femoral epiphysis, a further problem exists in that the normal hip joint is effectively lost, to be replaced by a false hip joint, or pseudarthrosis. This abnormal joint is more laterally placed, giving a reduced lever arm for the abductor muscles, and it may fail to provide the 'solid and stable fulcrum' required.

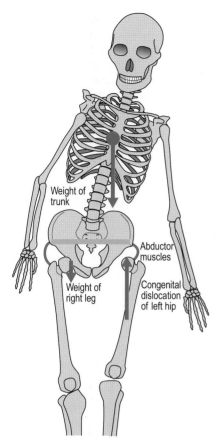

Fig. 3.5 • Congenital dislocation of the hip: both the working length and the lever arm of the hip abductors are reduced. To compensate, the subject bends the trunk over the supporting hip.

The combination of reduced lever arm and reduced muscle force gives these subjects a powerful incentive to walk with lateral trunk bending (Fig. 3.5). In many cases, particularly in older people with CDH, the false hip joint becomes arthritic and they add a painful hip to their other problems. Pain is frequently also a factor in slipped femoral epiphysis.

4. Wide walking base: If the walking base is abnormally wide, there is a problem with balance during single leg stance. Rather than tip the whole body to maintain balance, as in Figure 2.28A, lateral bending of the trunk may be used to keep the centre of gravity of the body roughly over the supporting leg. In most cases, this will need to be done during the stance phase on both sides, leading to bilateral trunk bending and a waddling gait. A number of conditions, which will be described later, may cause a wide walking base.

5. Unequal leg length: When walking with an unequal leg length, the pelvis tips downwards on the side of the shortened limb, as the body weight is transferred to it. This is sometimes described as 'stepping into a hole'. The pelvic tilt is accompanied by a compensatory lateral bend of the trunk.

6. Other causes: Perry (2010) gives a number of other causes for lateral bending of the trunk, including adductor contracture, scoliosis and an impaired body image, typically following a stroke.

Anterior trunk bending

In anterior trunk bending, the subject flexes his or her trunk forwards early in the stance phase. If only one leg is affected, the trunk is straightened again around the time of opposite initial contact, but if both sides are affected, the trunk may be kept flexed throughout the gait cycle. This gait abnormality is best seen from the side.

One important purpose of this gait pattern is to compensate for an inadequacy (weak) of the knee extensors. The left panel of Figure 3.6 shows that early in the stance phase, the line of action of the ground reaction force vector normally passes behind the axis of the knee joint and generates an external moment which attempts to flex it. This is opposed by contraction of the quadriceps, to generate an internal extension moment. If the quadriceps are weak or paralysed, they cannot generate this internal moment and the knee will tend to collapse. As shown in the

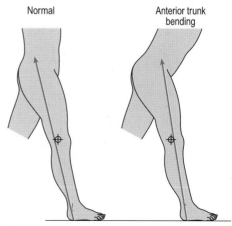

Fig. 3.6 • Anterior trunk bending: in normal walking, the line of force early in the stance phase passes behind the knee; anterior trunk bending brings the line of force in front of the knee, to compensate for weak knee extensors.

right panel of Figure 3.6, anterior trunk bending is used to move the centre of gravity of the body forwards, which results in the line of force passing in front of the axis of the knee, producing an external extension (or hyperextension) moment. In addition to anterior trunk bending, subjects will sometimes keep one hand on the affected thigh while walking, to provide further stabilisation for the knee.

Other causes for anterior trunk bending are equinus deformity of the foot, hip extensor weakness and hip flexion contracture (Perry, 2010).

Posterior trunk bending

One form of posterior trunk bending is essentially a reversed version of anterior trunk bending, in that early in the stance phase, the whole trunk moves in the sagittal plane, but this time backwards instead of forwards. Again, it is most easily observed from the side. The purpose of this is to compensate for ineffective (weak) hip extensors. The line of the ground reaction force early in the stance phase normally passes in front of the hip joint (Fig. 3.7, left panel). This produces an external moment which attempts to flex the trunk forward on the thigh and is opposed by contraction of the hip extensors, particularly the gluteus maximus. Should these muscles be weak or paralysed, the subject may compensate by moving the trunk backwards at this time, bringing the line of action of the external force behind the axis of the hip joint, as shown in the right panel diagram of Figure 3.7.

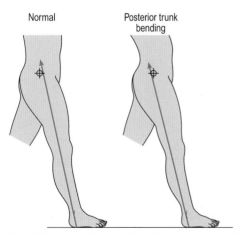

Normal   Posterior trunk bending

Fig. 3.7 • Posterior trunk bending: in normal walking, the line of force early in the stance phase passes in front of the hip; posterior trunk bending brings the line of force behind the hip, to compensate for weak hip extensors.

A different type of posterior trunk bending may occur early in the swing phase, where the subject may throw the trunk backwards in order to propel the swinging leg forwards. This is most often used to compensate for weakness of the hip flexors or spasticity of the hip extensors, either of which makes it difficult to accelerate the femur forwards at the beginning of swing. This manoeuvre may also be used if the knee is unable to flex, since the whole leg must be accelerated forwards as one unit, which greatly increases the demands on the hip flexors. Posterior trunk bending may also occur when the hip is ankylosed (fused), the trunk moving backwards as the thigh moves forwards.

Increased lumbar lordosis

Many people have an exaggerated lumbar lordosis, but it is only regarded as a gait abnormality if the lordosis is used to aid walking in some way, which generally means that the degree of lordosis varies during the course of the gait cycle. Increased lumbar lordosis is observed from the side of the subject and generally reaches a peak at the end of the stance phase on the affected side.

The most common cause of increased lumbar lordosis is a flexion contracture of the hip. It is also seen if the hip joint is immobile due to ankylosis. Both of these deformities cause the stride length to be very short, by preventing the femur from moving backwards from its flexed position. This difficulty can be overcome if the femur can be brought into the vertical (or even extended) position, not through movement at the hip joint but by extension of the lumbar spine, with a consequent increase in the lumbar lordosis (Fig. 3.8).

The orientation of the pelvis in the sagittal plane is maintained by the opposing pulls of the trunk muscles above and the limb muscles below. If there is muscle imbalance, for example a weakness of the muscles of the anterior abdominal wall, weakness of the hip extensors or spasticity of the hip flexors, the subject may develop an excessive *anterior pelvic tilt*, again with an increase in the lumbar lordosis.

Functional leg length discrepancy

Four gait abnormalities (circumduction, hip hiking, steppage and vaulting) are closely related, in that they are designed to overcome the same problem – a functional discrepancy in leg length. A review on

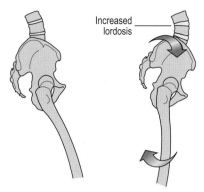

Fig. 3.8 • Increased lumbar lordosis: when there is a fixed flexion deformity of the hip (left panel), the whole pelvis must rotate forwards for the femur to move into a vertical position (right panel), with a resulting increase in lumbar lordosis.

the topic of leg length discrepancy was published by Gurney (2002).

An 'anatomical' leg length discrepancy occurs when the legs are actually different lengths, as measured with a tape measure or, more accurately, by long-leg X-rays. A 'functional' leg length discrepancy means that the legs are not necessarily different lengths (although they may be) but that one or both are unable to adjust to the appropriate length for a particular phase of the gait cycle. In order for natural walking to occur, the stance phase leg needs to be longer than the swing phase leg. If it is not, the swinging leg collides with the ground and is unable to pass the stance leg. The way that a leg is functionally lengthened (for the stance phase) is to extend at the hip and knee and to plantarflex at the ankle. Conversely, the way in which a leg is functionally shortened (for the swing phase) is to flex at the hip and knee and to dorsiflex at the ankle. Failure to achieve all the necessary flexions and extensions is likely to lead to a functional leg discrepancy and hence to one of these gait abnormalities. This usually occurs as the result of a neurological problem. Spasticity of any of the extensors or weakness of any of the flexors tends to make a leg too long in the swing phase, as does the mechanical locking of a joint in extension. Conversely, spasticity of the flexors, weakness of the extensors or a flexion contracture in a joint makes the limb too short for the stance phase. Other causes of functional leg length discrepancy include musculoskeletal problems such as sacroiliac joint dysfunction.

An increase in functional leg length is particularly common following a 'stroke', where a foot drop (due to anterior tibial weakness or paralysis) may be accompanied by an increase in tone in the hip and knee extensor muscles.

The gait modifications designed to overcome the problem may either lengthen the stance phase leg or shorten the swing phase leg, thus allowing a normal swing to occur. They are not mutually exclusive and a subject may use them in combination. The gait modification employed by a particular person may have been forced on them by the underlying pathology or it may have been a matter of chance. Two people with apparently identical clinical conditions may have found different solutions to the problem.

Circumduction

Ground contact by the swinging leg can be avoided if it is swung outward, in a movement known as circumduction (Fig. 3.9). The swing phase of the other leg will usually be normal. The movement of circumduction is best seen from in front or behind. Circumduction may also be used to advance the swinging leg in the presence of weak hip flexors, by improving the ability of the adductor muscles to act as hip flexors while the hip joint is extended.

Hip hiking

Hip hiking is a gait modification in which the pelvis is lifted on the side of the swinging leg (Fig. 3.10), by contraction of the spinal muscles and the lateral abdominal wall. The movement is best seen from behind or in front.

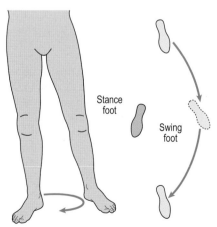

Fig. 3.9 • Circumduction: the swinging leg moves in an arc, rather than straight forwards, to increase the ground clearance for the swing foot.

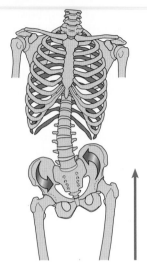

Fig. 3.10 • Hip hiking: the swing phase leg is lifted by raising the pelvis on that side.

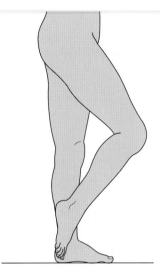

Fig. 3.11 • Steppage: increased hip and knee flexion improve ground clearance for the swing phase leg, in this case necessitated by a foot drop.

By tipping the pelvis up on the side of the swinging leg, hip hiking involves a reversal of the second determinant of gait (pelvic obliquity about an anteroposterior axis). It may also involve an exaggeration of the first determinant (pelvic rotation about a vertical axis), to assist with leg advancement. Leg advancement may also be helped by posterior trunk bending at the beginning of the swing phase.

According to the New York University manual (1986), hip hiking is commonly used in slow walking with weak hamstrings, since the knee tends to extend prematurely and thus to make the leg too long towards the end of the swing phase. It is seldom employed for limb lengthening due to plantarflexion of the ankle.

Steppage

Steppage is a very simple swing phase modification, consisting of exaggerated knee and hip flexion, to lift the foot higher than usual for increased ground clearance (Fig. 3.11). It is best observed from the side. It is particularly used to compensate for a plantarflexed ankle, commonly known as *foot drop*, due to inadequate dorsiflexion control, which will be described later.

Vaulting

The ground clearance for the swinging leg will be increased if the subject goes up on the toes of the stance phase leg, a movement known as vaulting

(Fig. 3.12). This causes an exaggerated vertical movement of the trunk, which is both ungainly in appearance and wasteful of energy. It may be observed from either the side or the front.

Vaulting is a stance phase modification, whereas the related gait abnormalities (circumduction, hip hiking and steppage) are swing phase modifications.

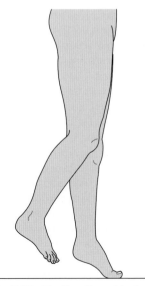

Fig. 3.12 • Vaulting: the subject goes up on the toes of the stance phase leg to increase ground clearance for the swing phase leg.

For this reason, vaulting may be a more appropriate solution for problems involving the swing phase leg. Like hip hiking, it is commonly used in slow walking with hamstring weakness, when the knee tends to extend too early in the swing phase. It may also be used on the 'normal' side of an above-knee amputee whose prosthetic knee fails to flex adequately in the swing phase.

Abnormal hip rotation

As the hip is able to make large rotations in the transverse plane, for which the knee and ankle cannot compensate, an abnormal rotation at the hip involves the whole leg, with the foot showing an abnormal 'toe in' or 'toe out' alignment. The gait pattern may involve both stance and swing phases and is best observed from behind or in front.

Abnormal hip rotation may result from one of three causes:

1. A problem with the muscles producing hip rotation

2. A fault in the way the foot makes contact with the ground

3. As a compensatory movement to overcome some other problem.

Problems with the muscles producing hip rotation usually involve spasticity or weakness of the muscles which rotate the femur about the hip joint. For example, overactivity of the medial hamstrings in cerebral palsy may include an element of internal rotation. Imbalance between the medial and lateral hamstrings is a common cause of rotation; weakness of biceps femoris or spasticity of the medial hamstrings will cause internal rotation of the leg. Conversely, spasticity of biceps femoris or weakness of the medial hamstrings will result in an external rotation.

A number of foot disorders will produce an abnormal rotation at the hip. Inversion of the foot, whether due to a fixed inversion (pes varus) or to weakness of the peroneal muscles, will internally rotate the whole limb when weight is taken on it. A corresponding eversion of the foot, whether fixed (pes valgus) or due to weakness of the anterior and posterior tibial muscles, will result in an external rotation of the hip.

External rotation may be used as a compensation for quadriceps weakness, to alter the direction of the line of force through the knee. This could be used as an alternative to, or in addition to, anterior trunk bending. External rotation may also be used to facilitate hip flexion, using the adductors as flexors, if the true hip flexors are weak. Subjects with weakness of the triceps surae may also externally rotate the leg, to permit the use of the peroneal muscles as plantar flexors. Femoral anteversion or retroversion could cause excessive hip internal or external rotation, respectively.

Excessive knee extension

In the gait abnormality of excessive knee extension, the normal stance phase flexion of the knee is lost, to be replaced by full extension or even hyperextension, in which the knee is angulated backwards. This is best seen from the side.

A few cause of knee hyperextension has already been described: quadriceps weakness can be compensated for by keeping the leg fully extended, using anterior trunk bending (Fig. 3.6), external rotation of the leg, or both, to keep the line of the ground reaction force from passing behind the axis of the knee joint. Other means of keeping the knee fully extended are pushing the thigh back by keeping one hand on it while walking and using the hip extensors to snap the thigh sharply back at the time of initial contact.

Hyperextension of the knee, accompanied by anterior trunk bending, is seen quite frequently in people with paralysis of the quadriceps following poliomyelitis. The gait abnormality is clearly of great value to the subject, since without it he or she would be unable to walk. However, the external hyperextension moment is resisted by tension in the posterior joint capsule, which gradually stretches, allowing the knee to develop a hyperextension deformity ('genu recurvatum'). As a result of this deformity, the joint frequently develops osteoarthritis in later life. This is illustrated in Figure 3.13, which shows the left sagittal plane hip, knee and ankle angles during walking in a 41-year-old woman, whose quadriceps were paralysed on both sides by poliomyelitis at the age of 12. She walked very slowly, using two forearm crutches (cycle time 1.9 s; cadence 63 steps/min; stride length 1.00 m; speed 0.52 m/s). The knee hyperextended to 32° during weightbearing, but flexed normally to 63° during the swing phase. The hip extended more than in normal individuals, since hyperextension of the knee places the knee joint more posteriorly than usual, thus altering the angle of the femur.

In normal walking, an external moment attempts to hyperextend the knee during terminal stance.

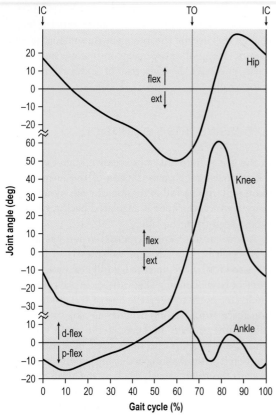

Fig. 3.13 • Excessive knee extension: sagittal plane hip, knee and ankle angles in a subject with paralysed quadriceps, showing gross hyperextension of the knee and increased extension of the hip. Abbreviations as in Figure 2.5.

the normal plantarflexion, and knee extension moments, which results in hyperextension of the knee.

Shortness of one leg may cause a person when standing to take all their weight on the other (longer) leg, with the knee hyperextended. This is because it is uncomfortable to stand on both legs, since the knee on the longer side would have to be kept flexed.

Excessive knee flexion

The knee is normally fully extended (or nearly so) twice during the gait cycle: around initial contact and around heel rise. In the gait abnormality known as excessive knee flexion, one or both of these movements into extension fails to occur. The flexion and extension of the knee are best seen from the side of the subject.

A flexion contracture of the knee will obviously prevent it from extending normally. A flexion contracture of the hip may also prevent the knee from extending, if hip flexion prevents the femur from becoming vertical or extended during the latter part of the stance phase (Fig. 3.14). By reducing the effective length of the leg during the stance phase, one of the compensations for a functional discrepancy in leg length will probably also be required.

Spasticity of the knee flexors may also cause the gait pattern of excessive knee flexion. Since the knee flexors are able to overpower the quadriceps, this

This is resisted by an internal flexor moment (see Fig. 2.6), generated primarily by gastrocnemius. Should gastrocnemius be weak, the knee may be pushed backwards into hyperextension. This may help with walking, since the leg lengthening required during pre-swing can be provided by extending the knee, rather than by plantarflexing the ankle. However, there is a risk that the knee will go beyond full extension into hyperextension, with consequent damage to the posterior capsule.

Hyperextension of the knee is common in spasticity. One common cause is overactivity of the quadriceps, which extends the knee directly. Another is spasticity of the triceps surae, which plantarflexes the ankle and causes the body weight to be taken through the forefoot. The resulting forward movement of the ground reaction force vector generates an external moment, which is an exaggeration of

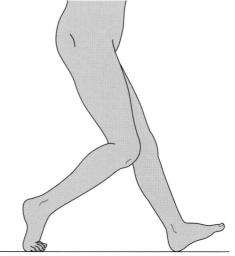

Fig. 3.14 • Excessive knee flexion: in late stance phase there is increased knee flexion, caused by a flexion contracture of the hip.

may lead to other gait modifications, such as anterior trunk bending, to compensate for a relative weakness of the quadriceps. The knee may flex excessively following initial contact if the normal plantarflexion of the foot during loading response is prevented, through immobility of the ankle joint or a calcaneus deformity of the foot, preventing the force vector from migrating forwards along the foot. Increased flexion of the knee may also be part of a compensatory movement, either to reduce the effective limb length in functional leg length discrepancy or as part of a pattern of exaggerated hip, knee and arm movements, to make up for a lack of plantarflexor power in push off.

Inadequate dorsiflexion control

The dorsiflexors are active at two different times during the gait cycle, so inadequate dorsiflexion control may give rise to two different gait abnormalities. During loading response, the dorsiflexors resist the external plantarflexion moment, thus permitting the foot to be lowered to the ground gently. If they are weak, the foot is lowered abruptly in a *foot slap*. The dorsiflexors are also active during the swing phase, when they are used to raise the foot and achieve ground clearance. Failure to raise the foot sufficiently during initial swing may cause *toe drag*. Both problems are best observed from the side of the subject and both make a distinctive noise. A subject with inadequate dorsiflexion control can often be diagnosed by ear, before they have come into view!

Inadequate dorsiflexion control may result from weakness or paralysis of the anterior tibial muscles or from these muscles being overpowered by spasticity of the triceps surae. An inability to dorsiflex the foot during the swing phase causes a functional leg length discrepancy, for which a number of compensations were described previously. Toe drag will only be observed if the subject fails to compensate. Toe drag may also occur if there is delayed flexion of the hip or knee in initial swing, causing the foot to catch on the ground, despite adequate dorsiflexion at the ankle.

Even if they suffer from inadequate dorsiflexion control, subjects with spasticity are frequently able to achieve dorsiflexion in the swing phase, because flexion of the hip and knee are often accompanied by reflex dorsiflexion of the ankle, in a primitive movement pattern related to the flexor withdrawal reflex, mentioned in Chapter 1.

Abnormal foot contact

The foot may be abnormally loaded so that the weight is primarily borne on only one of its four quadrants. Loading on the heel or forefoot is best observed from the side and loading on the medial or lateral side is best observed from the front, although some authorities state that the foot should always be observed from behind. Where a glass walkway is available, viewing the foot from below gives an excellent idea of the pattern of foot loading.

Loading of the heel occurs in the deformity known as *talipes calcaneus* (also known as pes calcaneus), where the forefoot is pulled up into extreme dorsiflexion (Fig. 3.15), usually as a result of muscle imbalance, such as results from spasticity of the anterior tibial muscles or weakness of the triceps surae. Except in mild cases, weight is never taken by the forefoot and the stance phase duration is reduced by the loss of the 'terminal rocker' (p. 75). The reduced stance phase duration on the affected side reduces the swing phase duration on the opposite side, which in turn reduces the opposite step length and the overall stride length. The ground reaction force vector remains posterior, producing an increased external flexion moment at the knee.

In the deformity known as *talipes equinus* (or pes equinus) (Fig. 3.16), the forefoot is fixed in plantarflexion, usually through spasticity of the plantarflexors. In a mild equinus deformity, the foot may be placed onto the ground flat; in more severe cases the heel never contacts the ground at all and initial contact is made by the metatarsal heads, in a gait pattern known as *primary toestrike*. Because the line of force from the ground reaction is displaced anteriorly, an increased external moment tending to extend the knee is present (plantarflexion/knee extension couple). The loss of the initial rocker (p. 55) shortens the stride length.

Excessive medial contact occurs in a number of foot deformities. Weakness of the inverters or

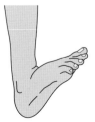

Fig. 3.15 • Talipes calcaneus.

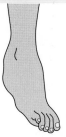

Fig. 3.16 • Talipes equinus.

spasticity of the everters will cause the medial side of the foot to drop and to take most of the weight. In *pes valgus*, the medial arch is lowered, permitting weightbearing on the medial border of the foot. Increased medial foot contact may also be due to a valgus deformity of the knee, accompanied by an increased walking base.

Excessive lateral foot contact may also result from foot deformity, when the medial border of the foot is elevated or the lateral border depressed, by spasticity or weakness. The foot deformity known as *talipes equinovarus* (Fig. 3.17) combines equinus with varus, producing a curved foot where all the load is borne by the outer border of the forefoot. Although the term *club foot* may be applied to any foot deformity, it is most commonly applied to talipes equinovarus.

Another form of abnormal foot contact is the *stamping* (walking with forcible steps) that commonly accompanies a loss of sensation in the foot, such as occurs in tabes dorsalis, the final stage of syphilis. The subject receives feedback on ground contact from the vibration caused by the impact of the foot on the ground.

Abnormal foot rotation

Normal individuals place the foot on the ground approximately in line with the direction of walk, typically with a few degrees of toe out. Pathological toe in or toe out angles may be produced by internal or external hip rotation, torsion (twisting) of the femur or tibia, or

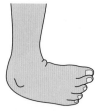

Fig. 3.17 • Talipes equinovarus.

deformity of the foot itself. An important consequence of an abnormal foot rotation is that it causes the ground reaction force to be in an abnormal position relative to the rest of the leg. For example, if the foot is internally rotated, the ground reaction force is more medial than normal, which will generate external adductor moments at the ankle and knee. In either internal or external foot rotation, the effective length of the foot is reduced in the direction of progression, so that the ground reaction force during terminal stance and pre-swing is likely to be more posterior than normal. This reduces the lever arm for the triceps surae to generate an internal plantarflexion moment.

This is one example of a problem known as *lever arm disease* or *lever arm deficiency*, in which individuals with normal muscle strength are unable to generate sufficient internal joint moments, due to a reduction in the length of a muscle's lever arm. This is particularly seen in individuals with cerebral palsy who have a severe degree of internal or external foot rotation; the resulting posterior placement of the ground reaction force increases the external moment flexing the knee.

Insufficient push off

In normal walking, weight is borne on the forefoot during the 'push off' in pre-swing. In the gait pattern known as insufficient push off, the weight is taken primarily on the heel and there is no push off phase, the whole foot being lifted off the ground at once. It is best observed from the side.

The main cause of insufficient push off is a problem with the triceps surae or Achilles tendon, which prevents adequate weightbearing on the forefoot. Rupture of the Achilles tendon and weakness of the soleus and gastrocnemius are typical causes. Weakness or paralysis of the intrinsic muscles of the foot may also prevent the foot from taking load through the forefoot. Insufficient push off may also result from any foot deformity, if the anatomy is so distorted that it prevents normal forefoot loading. A talipes calcaneus deformity (Fig. 3.15) obviously makes it impossible to put any significant load on the forefoot.

Another important cause of insufficient push off is pain under the forefoot, if the amount of pain is affected by the degree of loading (as it usually is). This may occur in metatarsalgia and also when arthritis affects the metatarsophalangeal joints. The loss of the terminal rocker causes the foot to leave the ground prematurely, before the hip has fully extended. This reduces the stance phase duration on the affected side and hence the swing phase duration and step length on the opposite side, and produces an asymmetry in gait timing.

Abnormal walking base

The walking base is usually in the range of 50–130 mm. In pathological gait it may be either increased or decreased beyond this range. While ideally determined by actual measurement, changes in the walking base may be estimated by eye, preferably from behind the subject.

An increased walking base may be caused by any deformity, such as an abducted hip or valgus knee, which causes the feet to be placed on the ground wider apart than usual. A consequence of an increased walking base is that increased lateral movement of the trunk is required to maintain balance, as shown in Figure 2.28.

The other important cause of an increased walking base is instability and a fear of falling, *which leads to the feet being placed wide apart to increase the area of support*. This allows a margin of error in the positioning of the centre of gravity over the feet. This gait abnormality is likely to be present when there is a deficiency in the sensation or proprioception of the legs, so that the subject is not quite sure where the feet are, relative to the trunk. It is also used in cerebellar ataxia, to increase the level of security in an uncoordinated gait pattern. Another effective way to improve stability is to walk with one or two canes.

A narrow walking base usually results from an adduction deformity at the hip or a varus deformity at the knee. Hip adduction may cause the swing phase leg to cross the midline, in a gait pattern known as *scissoring*, which is commonly seen in cerebral palsy. In milder cases, the swing phase leg is able to pass the stance phase leg, but then moves across in front of it. In more severe cases, the swinging leg is unable to pass the stance leg: it stops behind it, with the side-to-side positions of the two feet reversed. This is clearly a very disabling gait pattern, with a very short stride length and negative values for the walking base and for the step length on one side.

Rhythmic disturbances

Gait disorders may include abnormalities in the timing of the gait cycle. Two types of rhythmic disturbance can be identified: an *asymmetrical* rhythmic disturbance shows a difference in the gait timing between the two legs; an *irregular* rhythmic disturbance shows differences between one stride and the next. Rhythmic disturbances are best observed from the side and may also be audible.

An *antalgic* gait pattern is specifically a gait modification that reduces the amount of pain a person is experiencing. The term is usually applied to a rhythmic disturbance, in which as short a time as possible is spent on the painful limb and a correspondingly longer time is spent on the pain-free side. The pattern is *asymmetrical* between the two legs but is generally *regular* from one cycle to the next. A marked difference in leg length between the two sides may also produce a regular gait asymmetry of this type, as may a number of other differences between the two sides, such as joint contractures or ankylosis.

Irregular gait rhythmic disturbances, where the timing alters from one step to the next, are seen in a number of neurological conditions. In particular, cerebellar ataxia leads to loss of the 'pattern generator', responsible for a regular, coordinated sequence of footsteps. Loss of sensation or proprioception may also cause an irregular arrhythmia, due to a general uncertainty about limb position and orientation.

Other gait abnormalities

A number of other gait abnormalities may be observed, either alone or in combination with some of the gait patterns described above. They include:

1. Abnormal movements, for example intention tremors and athetoid movements
2. Abnormal attitude or movements of the upper limb, including a failure to swing the arms
3. Abnormal attitude or movements of the head and neck
4. Sideways rotation of the foot following heelstrike
5. Excessive external rotation of the foot during swing, sometimes called a 'whip'
6. Rapid fatigue.

This account has concentrated on gait abnormalities which may be observed visually. However, a number of gait abnormalities can only be detected using kinetic/kinematic gait analysis systems. An example is the presence of an abnormal moment, such as the excessive internal varus moment which may be present in the knee of children with myelomeningocoele and which may predispose them to the development of osteoarthritis (Lim et al., 1998).

Walking aids

The use of walking aids may modify the gait pattern considerably. While some people choose to use a walking aid to make it easier to walk, for example to reduce the pain in a painful joint, others are totally unable to walk without some form of aid. Although there are many detailed variations in design, walking aids, also called 'assistive devices', can be classified into three basic types – *canes*, *crutches* and *frames*. All three operate by supporting part of the body weight through the arm rather than the leg. While this is an effective way of coping with inadequacies of the legs, it frequently leads to problems with the wrist and shoulder joints, which are simply not designed for the transmission of large forces.

There is considerable variability in the way in which walking aids are used and people will often use them in ways which do not quite fit the typical patterns described in the following sections.

Canes

The simplest form of walking aid is the cane, also known as a walking stick, by means of which force can be transmitted to the ground through the wrist and hand. Since the forearm muscles are relatively weak and the joints of the wrist fairly small, it is impossible to transmit large forces through a cane for any length of time. The torque which can be applied to the upper end of the cane is limited by the grip strength and by the shape of the handle, since the hand tends to slip. For this reason the major direction of force transmission is along the axis of the cane. Canes may be used for three purposes, which are often combined:

1. To improve stability
2. To generate a moment
3. To take part of the load away from one of the legs.

Improve stability

Canes are frequently used by elderly and infirm people to improve their stability. This is achieved by increasing the size of the area of support, thus removing the need to position the centre of gravity over the relatively small supporting area provided by the feet. In those with only minor stability problems, a single cane may be used. This will not provide a secure supporting area during single limb support, but does make it easier to correct for small imbalances. Since

the cane is usually placed on the ground some distance away from the feet, giving a relatively long lever arm, a modest force through the cane will produce a substantial moment to correct for any positioning error. For maximum security, a person will need to use two canes, so that a triangular supporting area is always available. This is provided by two canes and one foot during single limb support and by one cane and two feet during double support. If only a single cane is used, it will usually be advanced during the stance phase of the more secure leg. If two canes are used, they are usually advanced separately, during double limb support, to provide the maximum stability at all times.

Generate a moment

The use of a cane to generate a moment is illustrated in Figure 3.18. A vertical force of 100 N (10 kgf or 22 lbf) is applied through the cane, which generates a clockwise moment, applied to the shoulder girdle and hence to the pelvis. This reduces the size of the moment which the hip abductor muscles need to generate to keep the pelvis level. The contraction of these muscles is reduced from 911 N (93 kgf or 204 lbf) to 463 N (47 kgf or 104 lbf), a reduction of 448 N (56 kgf or 123 lbf). The total force in the hip joint is reduced by the sum of this amount and the force applied by the cane to the ground. For this mechanism to work, the cane must be held in the opposite hand to the painful hip. A cane may also be used to generate a lateral moment at the knee, to reduce the loading on one side of the joint. The cane is advanced during the swing phase of the leg it is protecting.

Reduce limb loading

When using a cane to remove some of the load from the leg, it is usually held in the same hand as the affected leg and placed on the ground close to the foot. In this way, load sharing can be achieved between the leg and the cane, even to the extent of removing the load entirely from the leg. The cane follows the movements of the affected leg, being advanced during the swing phase on that side. The person will normally lean sideways over the cane, in a lateral lurch, to increase the vertical loading on it and hence to reduce the load in the leg. A cane may be used in this way to relieve pain in the hip, knee, ankle or foot. If the cane is held in the opposite hand, as is often recommended, the lateral lurching can be avoided but the degree of off-loading is reduced.

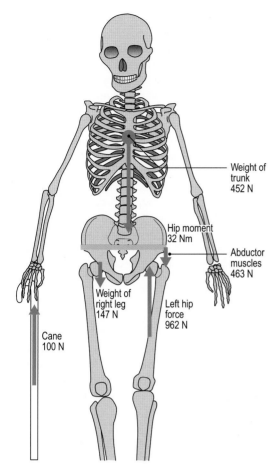

Fig. 3.18 • The use of a cane to generate a clockwise moment reduces the contraction force of the hip abductors and hence the force in the hip joint, during right leg swing phase. The force in the left hip (962 N) is the sum of: (i) weight of trunk (452 N), (ii) weight of right leg (147 N), (iii) contraction force of abductor muscles (463 N), less: (iv) force through cane (100 N). (Compare with Figure 3.2 (force in left hip of 1510 N during single leg stance).)

Whichever of these three reasons a person has for using a cane, the degree of disability will determine whether one or two canes are used. It may be observed that a subject uses a cane in the opposite hand from what might have been expected. In some cases he or she has simply not discovered that they would benefit more from using the cane in the other hand but more often, the observer has failed to appreciate fully all the compensations which the subject has adopted.

There are a number of ways in which the simple cane can be modified, including many different types of handgrip. A particularly important variant on the simple cane is the *broad based cane*, also known as a *Hemi* or *crab cane*, which may have three feet (*tripod*) or four feet (*tetrapod* or *quad cane*). This differs from the simple cane in that it will stand up by itself and will tolerate small horizontal force components, so long as the overall force vector remains within the area of its base. It is particularly helpful when standing up from the sitting position. The increased stability is gained at the expense of an increase in weight and particularly bulk, which may cause difficulties when going through doorways.

Crutches

The main difference in function between a crutch and a cane is that a crutch is able to transmit significant forces in the horizontal plane. This is because, unlike the cane, which is effectively fixed to the body at only a single point, the crutch has two points of attachment, one at the hand and one higher up the arm, which provide a lever arm for the transmission of torque. Although there are many different designs of crutch, they fall into two categories: axillary crutches and forearm crutches. As with the cane, it is also possible to have a broad-based crutch, ending in three or four feet.

Axillary crutches (Fig. 3.19, left panel), as their name suggests, fit under the axilla (armpit). They

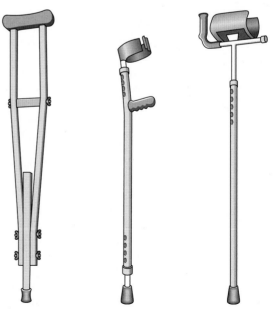

Fig. 3.19 • Three types of crutches: axillary (left); forearm (centre) and gutter (right).

are usually of simple design, with a padded top surface and a hand-hold in the appropriate position. The lever arm between the axilla and the hand is fairly long and enough horizontal force can be generated to permit walking when both legs are straight and non-functional. A disadvantage of this type of crutch is that the axilla is not an ideal area for weight-bearing and incorrect fitting or prolonged use may damage the blood vessels or nerves. Although some people use axillary crutches for many years, they are more suitable for short-term use, for instance while a patient has a broken leg set in plaster.

There are many different types of *forearm crutches*, also called *elbow*, *Lofstrand* or *Canadian crutches* (Fig. 3.19, middle panel). They differ from axillary crutches in that the upper point of contact between the body and the crutch is provided by either the forearm or the upper arm, rather than by the axilla. The lever arm is thus shorter than for an axillary crutch, although this is seldom a problem, and they usually run less risk of tissue damage, as well as being lighter and more acceptable cosmetically. In the normal forearm crutch, most of the vertical force is transmitted through the hand, but the use of a 'gutter' or 'platform' permits more load to be taken by the forearm itself (Fig. 3.19, right panel).

Walking frames

The most stable walking aid is the frame, also called a 'walker' or 'Zimmer frame', which enables the subject to stand and walk within the area of support provided by its base. Considerable force can be applied to the frame vertically and moderate forces can be applied horizontally, provided that the overall force vector remains within the area of support. The usual method of walking is first to move the frame forwards, then to take a short step with each foot, then to move the frame again, and so on. Walking is thus extremely slow, with a start-stop pattern. Although the subject is encouraged to lift the frame forward at each step, they are more often simply slid along the ground.

A *rolling walker* is a variant on the walking frame, in which the front feet are replaced by wheels. This makes it easier to advance, at the expense of a slight reduction in stability in the direction of progression. The mode of walking is very similar to that with the frame, except that it is easier to move forwards, since tipping the rolling walker lifts the back feet clear of the ground. Commonly patients misuse

the rolling walker by sliding it forwards, rather than tipping it and tennis balls are now frequently placed on the rear legs to facilitate sliding it due to its frequent occurrence. A further variant on the design is a *rollator*, which is a walking frame that has four wheels on all four legs, and is equipped with hand-operated brakes. These devices also often have seats in the middle, which the operator can use if they need to quickly sit, but the operator must turn around and face the opposite direction before sitting in most models. There are many other designs of frames and walkers, including those which fold, those with 'gutters' to support the body weight through the forearms, and those in which the two sides are connected at the back, rather than at the front. The stop–start gait pattern seen with some walking aids (especially frames) is known as an 'arrest gait'.

Gait patterns with walking aids

There are a number of different ways of walking when using a cane, crutch or walker. The terminology varies somewhat from one author to another; the descriptions which follow are based on the well-illustrated text by Pierson (1994). The first four gait patterns involve the greatest support from the upper limbs, by means of a walking frame, two crutches or two canes. The last two require less support, with a crutch or cane held in only one hand.

1. Four-point gait can be employed with canes or crutches. Also known as 'reciprocal gait', it involves the separate and alternate movement of each of the two legs and the two walking aids, for example: left crutch – right leg – right crutch – left leg (Fig. 3.20). This pattern is very stable and requires little energy but it is very slow, so that the oxygen cost (oxygen consumption per unit distance) may be higher than for the three-point gait described below.

2. Three-point gait is used when only one leg can take weight or the two legs move together as a single unit. It is only used with crutches or a walker. Two main forms of three-point gait are recognised: *step-through* and *step-to*. These terms are used when the lower limb musculature is able to provide the movement of the legs. If the legs are paralysed and their movement is provided by the upper limbs and trunk, the terms *swing-through* and *swing-to* are used (Pierson, 1994). In step-through gait, the foot or feet move from behind

Fig. 3.20 • Four-point gait. One crutch or leg is moved at a time in the pattern: left crutch – right leg – right crutch – left leg.

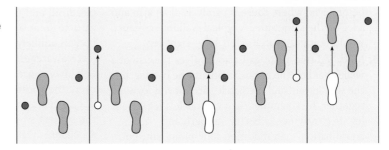

the line of the two crutches to in front of them (Fig. 3.21). This gait pattern requires a lot of energy and good control of balance but it can be fairly fast. In step-to gait, the foot or feet are advanced to just behind the line of the crutches, which are then moved further forwards and the process repeated (Fig. 3.22). Since the stride length is short, walking speed is slow but energy and stability requirements are not as high as for step-through gait.

3. Modified three-point gait (also known as *three-one gait*) may be used when one leg is able to take full body weight but the other is not. It may be employed with a walker or with two crutches or canes. The walking aids and the affected leg move forward together, while weight is taken on the sound leg. That leg is then advanced, while weight is taken on the bad leg and the walking aids. This makes for a stable gait pattern, requiring little strength or energy, but the speed is fairly low.

4. Two-point gait resembles four-point gait, except that the crutch or cane on one side is moved forward at the same time as the leg on the other, for example: left crutch/right leg – right crutch/ left leg. It is faster than four-point gait, yet is still fairly stable and requires little energy. However, it demands good coordination by the subject.

5. Modified four-point gait is performed when the walking aid is carried in the opposite hand to the affected leg. This gait pattern is typically used in

Fig. 3.21 • Three-point step-through gait in a person taking weight on both legs. The legs are advanced together, in front of the line of the crutches, then the crutches are advanced together, in front of the line of the legs.

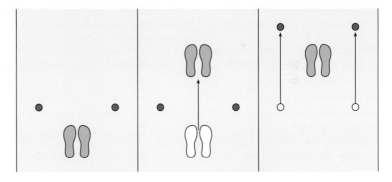

Fig. 3.22 • Three-point step-to gait in a person taking weight on only one leg. The leg is advanced to behind the line of the crutches, which are then moved forwards again.

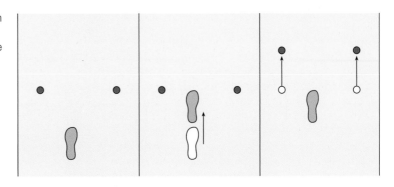

hemiplegia, where there is paralysis of an arm and a leg on the same side. A typical walking sequence would be right crutch – left leg – right leg.

6. Modified two-point gait also involves the use of a walking aid on the opposite side to the bad leg, but the walking aid and the bad leg are moved forward together, for example: right crutch/left leg – right leg. It clearly needs better strength and coordination than modified four-point gait, but gives better speed.

Treadmill gait

It is often more convenient to study gait while the subject walks on a treadmill rather than over the ground, since the volume in which measurements need to be made is much smaller and they can conveniently be connected to wires or breathing tubes. However, there are subtle differences between treadmill and overground gait, particularly with regard to joint angles. The reduced airflow over the body is unlikely to be a significant factor, but the subject's awareness of the limited length of the treadmill belt may cause them to shorten their stride. However, the most important differences are probably due to changes in the speed of the treadmill belt, as the subject's feet decelerate it at initial contact and accelerate it at push off, effectively storing energy in the treadmill motor. This effect is minimised by using a large treadmill with a powerful motor (Savelberg et al., 1998). Treadmills instrumented with force plates have been used to examine potential differences between overground and treadmill walking and running. In general, these studies have found minimal differences in treadmill walking/running versus overground walking/running in both kinetic and kinematic parameters, provided the treadmill belt was sufficiently stiff and that subjects were acclimated to treadmill use (Riley et al., 2008).

References

Gurney, B., 2002. Leg length discrepancy. Gait Posture 15, 195–206.

Lim, R., Dias, L., Vankoski, S., et al., 1998. Valgus knee stress in lumbosacral myelomeningocele: a gait-analysis evaluation. J. Pediatr. Orthop. 18, 428–433.

New York University, 1986. Lower Limb Orthotics. New York University Postgraduate Medical School, New York, NY.

Perry, J., 2010. Gait Analysis: Normal and Pathological Function. Slack Incorporated, Thorofare, NJ.

Pierson, F.M., 1994. Principles and Techniques of Patient Care. WB Saunders, Philadelphia, PA.

Riley, P.O., Paolini, G., Croce, U.D., et al., 2008. A kinematics and kinetic comparison of overground and treadmill running. Med. Sci. Sports Exerc. 40 (6), 1093–1100.

Savelberg, H.H.C.M., Vorstenbosch, M.A.T.M., Kamman, E.H., et al., 1998. Intra-stride belt-speed variation affects treadmill locomotion. Gait Posture 7, 26–34.

Further reading

Saunders, J.B.D.M., Inman, V.T., Eberhart, H.S., 1953. The major determinants in normal and pathological gait. J. Bone Joint Surg. Am. 35, 543–558.

Methods of gait analysis

4

Michael Whittle   David Levine   Jim Richards

Walking is often impaired by neurological and musculoskeletal pathology and is one of the health domains of the International Classification of Functioning, Disability and Health (ICF). It is a key aspect in the activities and participation component for mobility and is often adopted as the underlying framework for the assessment of mobility in clinical practice. Therefore it is very important for members of an interdisciplinary team to assess any loss of function in gait.

Gait analysis is used for two very different purposes: to aid directly in the treatment of individual patients and to improve our understanding of gait through research. Gait research use may be further subdivided into 'fundamental' studies of walking and clinical research. These topics are explored further in the next chapter. Clearly, no single method of analysis is suitable for such a wide range of uses and a number of different methodologies have been developed.

When considering the methods which may be used to perform gait analysis, it is helpful to regard them as being in a 'spectrum' or 'continuum', ranging from the absence of technological aids, at one extreme, to the use of complicated and expensive equipment at the other. This chapter starts with a method which requires no equipment at all and goes on to describe progressively more elaborate systems. As a general rule, the more elaborate the system, the higher the cost, but the better the quality of objective data that can be provided. However, this does not imply that some of the simpler techniques are not worth using. It has often been found, particularly in a clinical setting, that the use of high-technology gait analysis is inappropriate, because of its high cost

in terms of money, space and time, and because some clinical problems can be adequately managed using simpler techniques.

Visual gait analysis

It is tempting to say that the simplest form of gait analysis is that made by the unaided human eye. This, of course, neglects the remarkable abilities of the human brain to process the data received by the eye. Visual gait analysis is, in reality, the most complicated and versatile form of analysis available. Despite this, it suffers from serious limitations:

1. It is transitory, giving no permanent record
2. The eye cannot observe high-speed events
3. It is only possible to observe movements, not forces
4. It depends entirely on the skill of the individual observer
5. It is subjective and it can be difficult to avoid assessor bias if the patient is undergoing treatment
6. Subjects may act differently when they know they are being watched (Hawthorne effect)
7. A clinic or laboratory environment may be very different than the real world.

In a study on the reproducibility of visual gait analysis, Krebs et al. (1985) found it to be 'only moderately reliable'. Saleh and Murdoch (1985) compared the performance of people skilled in visual gait analysis with the data provided by a combined kinetic/kinematic system. They found that the measurement system identified many more gait abnormalities than had been seen by the observers.

Many clinicians include the observation of a subject's gait as part of their clinical examination. However, this is not gait analysis if it is limited to watching the subject make a single walk, up and down the room. This merely gives a superficial idea of how well they walk and perhaps identifies the most serious abnormality. A thorough visual gait analysis involves watching the subject while he or she makes a number of walks, some of which are observed from one side, some from the other side, some from the front and some from the back. As the subject walks, the observer should look for the presence or absence of a number of specific gait abnormalities, such as those described in Chapter 3 and summarised in Table 4.1. A logical order should be used for looking for the different gait abnormalities – the mixture of walking directions listed in the table is not recommended! According to Rose (1983), it is also important, when performing visual gait analysis, to compare the ranges of motion at the joints during walking with those which are observed on the examination plinth – they may be either greater or smaller.

The minimum length required for a gait analysis walkway is a hotly debated subject. The authors believe that 8 m (26 ft) is about the minimum for use with fit young people, but that at least 12 m (39 ft) is preferable, since it permits fast walkers to 'get into their stride' before any measurements are made. However, shorter walkways are satisfactory for people who walk more slowly. This particularly applies to those with a pathological gait, since the gait pattern usually stabilises within the first two or three steps. A notable exception to this, however, is the gait in parkinsonism, which 'evolves' over the first few strides. The width required for a walkway depends on what equipment, if any, is being used to make measurements. For visual gait analysis, as little as 3 m (10 ft) may be sufficient. If video recording is being used, the camera needs to be positioned a little further from the subject and about 4 m (13 ft) is needed. A kinematic system making simultaneous measurements from both sides of the body normally requires a width of at least 5–6 m (16–20 ft). Figure 4.1 shows the layout of a small gait laboratory used for visual gait analysis, video recording and the measurement of the general gait parameters.

Some investigators permit subjects to choose their own walking speed, whereas others control the cycle time (number of steps in a set time) or the cadence (steps per minute), for example by asking them to walk in time with a metronome. The rationale for controlling the cadence is that many of the measurable parameters of gait vary with the walking speed and controlling this provides one means of reducing the variability. However, subjects are unlikely to walk naturally when trying to keep pace with a metronome, and patients with motor control problems may find it difficult or even impossible to walk at an imposed cadence. Zijlstra et al. (1995) found considerable differences in the gait of normal subjects between 'natural' walking and 'constrained' walking, in which the subject was required either to step in time with a metronome or to step on particular places on the ground. The answer to this dilemma is probably to accept the fact that subjects need to walk at different speeds and to interpret the data appropriately. This means that 'normal' values must be available for a range of walking speeds. An unresolved difficulty with this approach is that it may not be possible to get 'normal' values for very slow walking speeds, since normal individuals do not customarily

Table 4.1 Common gait abnormalities and best direction for observation

Gait abnormality	Observing direction
Lateral trunk bending	Side
Anterior trunk bending	Side
Posterior trunk bending	Side
Increased lumbar lordosis	Side
Circumduction	Front or behind
Hip hiking	Front or behind
Steppage	Side
Vaulting	Side or front
Abnormal hip rotation	Front or behind
Excessive knee extension	Side
Excessive knee flexion	Side
Inadequate dorsiflexion control	Side
Abnormal foot contact	Front or behind
Abnormal foot rotation	Front or behind
Insufficient push off	Side
Abnormal walking base	Front or behind
Rhythmic disturbances	Side

Fig. 4.1 • Layout of a small gait laboratory for visual gait analysis, video recording and measurement of the general gait parameters.

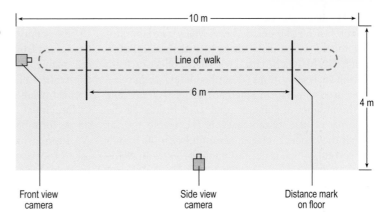

walk very slowly and when asked to do so, some of the gait measurements become very variable (Brandstater et al., 1983).

Gait assessment

Simply observing the gait and noting abnormalities is of little value by itself. It needs to be followed by gait assessment, which is the synthesis of these observations with other information about the subject, obtained from the history and physical examination, combined with the intelligence and experience of the observer (Rose, 1983). Visual gait analysis is entirely subjective and the quality of the analysis depends on the skill of the person performing it. It can be an interesting exercise to perform visual gait analysis on people walking past in the street, but without knowing their clinical details it is easy to misinterpret what is wrong with them.

When performing any type of gait analysis, one thing that must be constantly borne in mind is that you are observing effects and not causes. Putting it another way, the observed gait pattern is not the direct result of a pathological process but the net result of a pathological process and the subject's attempts to compensate for it. The observed gait pattern is 'what is left after the available mechanisms for compensation have been exhausted' (Rose, 1983).

Examination by video recording

Historically the use of videotape was widespread in the 1990s, although now this is achieved by direct recording to a DVD, memory card or computer. This has provided one of the most useful enhancements to gait analysis in the clinical setting during recent years. This helps to overcome two of the limitations of visual gait analysis: the lack of a permanent record and the difficulty of observing high-speed events. In addition, it confers the following advantages:

1. It reduces the number of walks a subject needs to do
2. It makes it possible to show the subject exactly how they are walking
3. It makes it easier to teach visual gait analysis to someone else
4. It completes the picture in a gait report as seeing the patient is very meaningful while reading values of their analysis.

Gait examination by video recording is not an objective method, since it does not provide quantitative data in the form of numbers. However, it does provide a permanent record, which can be extremely valuable. The presence of an earlier recording of a subject's gait may be used to demonstrate to all concerned how much progress has been made, especially when this has occurred over a long period of time. In particular, it may convince a subject or family member that an improvement *has* occurred, when memory tells them that they are no better than they were several months ago!

When using video recording, the most practical system consists of camcorder(s). The majority of today's domestic camcorders are perfectly suitable for use in gait analysis, the requirements being a zoom lens, automatic focus, the ability to operate in normal room lighting and an electronically shuttered charge-coupled device (CCD) sensor, to eliminate blurring due to movement. These allow the user to freeze-frame the picture and to advance frame by frame through successive frames, or to play at a very slow speed to allow the user to observe movements which are too fast for the unaided eye. Many gait laboratories record video data directly into a computer, which may be synchronised with data collection from motion analysis systems (described later), or in some cases used to perform kinematic analysis depending on the number of cameras used. One limitation the majority of camcorders have is the frame rate at which they collect images, commonly 25–30 frames per second, which is not fast enough to pick up some subtleties of movement. However, with the correct software, it is possible to obtain a maximum sampling rate of 50 Hz for PAL (Phase Alternating Line) and 60 Hz for NTSC (National Television Standards Committee) based systems and new developments in video technology include lower cost, higher speed cameras.

In making a thorough visual gait analysis without the use of video recording, the subject needs to make repeated walks to confirm or refute the presence of each of the gait abnormalities listed in Table 4.1. If the subject is in pain or easily fatigued, this may be an unreasonable requirement and it may be difficult to achieve a satisfactory analysis. The use of video recording permits the subject to do a much smaller number of walks, as the person performing the analysis can watch the recording as many times as necessary.

Video recording facilitates the process of teaching visual gait analysis, in which the student often needs to see small abnormal movements which happen very quickly. It is much easier to see such movements if the gait can be examined in slow motion, with the instructor pointing out details on the television or computer monitor. The use of video recording also makes it possible to observe a variety of abnormal gaits which have been archived. A number of teaching animations are now available (Appendix 3).

Showing the subject a video recording of their own gait is not exactly 'biofeedback', since there is a time delay involved, but nonetheless it can be very helpful. When a therapist is working with a subject to correct a gait abnormality, the subject may gain a clearer idea of exactly what the therapist is concerned about if they can observe their own gait from the 'outside'.

Although visual gait analysis using video recording is subjective, it is easy, at the same time, to derive some objective data. The general gait parameters (cycle time or cadence, stride length and speed) can be measured by a method which will be described in the next section. It is also possible to measure joint angles by using some form of on-screen digitiser such as

Siliconcoach and Dartfish. Such measurements tend to be susceptible to some errors as the joints may not be viewed from precisely the correct angle, although reasonable joint movements of the lower limb in the sagittal plane and some joint movements in the coronal plane can be obtained.

Individual investigators will find their own ways of performing gait analysis using video recording. A common routine used involves the subject being asked to wear shorts or a swim suit, so that the majority of the leg is visible. It is important that the subject should walk as 'normally' as possible, so they are asked to wear their own indoor or outdoor shoes, with socks if preferred. Unless it would unduly tire the subject, it is a good idea to make one or two 'practice' walks, before starting video recording. Two camera positions are often used, one viewing from the side (sagittal plane) and the front (coronal plane) (Fig. 4.1). These are first adjusted to show the whole body from head to feet and the subject is recorded as they walk the length of the walkway in one direction. At the end of the walkway, the subject turns around, with a rest if necessary, and is recorded as they walk back again. The whole process may then be repeated with the cameras adjusted to show a close-up of the body from the waist down, or of the body segment of interest.

It is often helpful to mark the subject's skin, for example using an eyebrow pencil or whiteboard marker, to enhance the visibility of anatomical landmarks on the recording. Hillman et al. (1998) fitted subjects with surface-mounted 'rotation indicators', to improve the accuracy with which transverse plane rotations were estimated from video recording.

Subjects should not be able to see themselves on a monitor while they are walking, as this provides a distraction, particularly for children. The cameras should also be placed in a manner so that they are not a focus point. Whether they are shown the video recording afterwards is at the discretion of the investigator, although it is important to review the recording before the subject leaves, in case it needs to be repeated for some reason.

The analysis is performed by replaying the video recording, looking for specific gait abnormalities in the different views and interpreting what is seen in the light of the subject's history and physical examination. It is particularly helpful if two or more people work together to perform the analysis. Rose (1983) suggested that gait analysis should be based on the team approach, with discussion and hypothesis testing. As will be described in Chapter 5, hypothesis testing may involve an attempted modification of the gait, for instance by fitting an orthosis or by paralysing a muscle using local anaesthesia.

Temporal and spatial parameters during gait

Temporal and spatial parameters of gait, sometimes referred to as the general gait parameters, include cycle time (or stride time), stride length and speed. These provide the simplest form of objective gait evaluation (Robinson and Smidt, 1981) and may be made using only a stopwatch and a tape measure. Other temporal and spatial parameters of gait include, step time, double support time, single support time, step length, base width and foot angle. However these measurements require the use of specialist equipment which will be described in the next section.

Cycle time, stride length and speed tend to change together in most locomotor disabilities, so that a subject with a long cycle time will usually also have a short stride length and a low speed (speed being stride length divided by cycle time). The general gait parameters give a guide to the walking ability of a subject, but little specific information. They should always be interpreted in terms of the expected values for the subject's age and sex, such as those covered in Chapter 2. Figure 4.2 shows one way in which these data may be presented; the diamonds represent the

95% confidence limits for a normal subject of the same age and sex as the subject under investigation. Although cycle time is gradually replacing cadence in the gait analysis community, it is more convenient to use cadence on plots of this type, since abnormally slow gait will give values on the left-hand side of the graph for all three of the general gait parameters.

Cycle time or cadence

Cycle time or cadence may be measured with the aid of a stopwatch, by counting the number of individual steps taken during a known period of time. It is seldom practical to count for a full minute, so a period of 10 or 15 seconds is usually chosen. The loss of accuracy incurred by counting for such short periods of time is unlikely to be of any practical significance. The subject should be told to walk naturally and they should be allowed to get up to their full walking speed before the observer starts to count the steps. The cycle time is calculated using the formula:

$$\text{cycle time (s)} = \text{time (s)} \times 2/\text{steps counted}$$

The number '2' allows for the fact that there are two steps per stride. The cadence is calculated using the formula:

$$\text{cadence (steps/min)} = \text{steps counted} \times 60/\text{time (s)}$$

The number '60' allows for the fact that there are 60 seconds in a minute.

Stride length

Stride length can be determined in two ways: by direct measurement or indirectly from the speed and cycle time. The simplest direct method of measurement is to count the strides taken while the subject covers a known distance. More useful methods include putting ink pads on the soles of the subject's shoes and walking on paper (Rafferty and Bell, 1995), using marker pens attached to shoes (Gerny, 1983) and a more messy option is to have the subject step with both feet in a shallow tray of talcum powder and then walk across a polished floor or along a strip of brown wrapping paper or coloured 'construction paper', leaving a trail of footprints. These may be measured, as shown in Figure 2.3, to derive left and right step lengths, stride length, walking base, toe out angle and some idea of the foot contact pattern. This investigation is able to provide

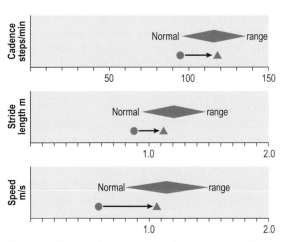

Fig. 4.2 • Display of the general gait parameters, with normal ranges appropriate for a patient's age and sex. Pre- and postoperative values for a 70-year-old female patient undergoing knee replacement surgery.

a great deal of useful and surprisingly accurate information, for the sake of a few minutes of mopping up the floor afterwards! As an alternative to using talcum powder, felt adhesive pads, soaked in different coloured dyes, may be fixed to the feet (Rose, 1983). The subject walks along a strip of paper and leaves a pattern of dots, which give an accurate indication of the locations of both feet.

If both the cycle time and the speed have been measured, stride length may be calculated using the formula:

$$\text{stride length (m)} = \text{speed (m/s)} \times \text{cycle time (s)}$$

The equivalent calculation using cadence is:

$$\text{stride length (m)} = \frac{\text{speed (m/s)} \times 2 \times 60}{\text{cadence (steps/min)}}$$

The multiplication by '2' converts steps to strides and by '60' converts minutes to seconds. For accurate results, the cycle time and speed should be measured during the same walk. However, the simultaneous counting, measuring and timing may prove too difficult and the errors introduced by using data from different walks are not likely to be important, unless the subject's gait varies markedly from one walk to another.

Speed

The speed may be measured by timing the subject while he or she walks a known distance, for example between two marks on the floor or between two pillars in a corridor. The distance walked is a matter of convenience but somewhere in the region of 6–10 m (20–33 ft) is probably adequate. Again, the subject should be told to walk at their natural speed and they should be allowed to get into their stride before the measurement starts. The speed is calculated as follows:

$$\text{speed (m/s)} = \text{distance (m)/time (s)}$$

General gait parameters from video recording

Determination of the general gait parameters from a video recording of the subject walking is easy, providing the recording shows the subject passing two landmarks whose positions are known. One simple method is to have the subject walk across two lines on the floor, a known distance apart, made with adhesive tape. Space should be allowed for acceleration before the first line and for slowing down after the second one. When the recording is replayed, the time taken to cover the distance is measured and the steps taken are counted. It is easiest to take the first initial contact *beyond the start line* as the point to begin both timing and counting and the first initial contact *beyond the finish line* as the point to end both timing and counting. The first step beyond the start line must be counted as 'zero', not 'one'. This method of measurement is not strictly accurate, since the position of the foot at initial contact is an unknown distance beyond the start and finish line, but the errors introduced are unlikely to be significant. As mentioned above, this method can also be employed without the use of video recording.

Since the distance, the time and the number of steps are all known, the general gait parameters can be calculated using the formulae:

$$\text{cycle time (s)} = \text{time (s)} \times 2/\text{steps counted}$$
$$\text{cadence (steps/min)} = \text{steps counted} \times 60/\text{time (s)}$$
$$\text{stride length (m)} = \text{distance (m)} \times 2/\text{steps counted}$$
$$\text{speed (m/s)} = \text{distance (m)/time (s)}$$

Measurement of temporal and spatial parameters during gait

A number of systems have been described which perform the automatic measurement of the timing of the gait cycle, sometimes called the temporal gait parameters. Such systems may be divided into two main classes: footswitches and instrumented walkways. Figure 4.3 shows typical data, which could be obtained from either type of system.

Footswitches

Footswitches are used to record the timing of gait. If one switch is fixed beneath the heel and one beneath the forefoot, it is possible to measure the timing of initial contact, foot flat, heel rise and toe off, and the duration of the stance phase (see Figs 2.2 and 4.3). Data from two or more strides make it possible to calculate cycle time and swing phase duration. If switches are mounted on both feet, the single and double support times can also be measured. The footswitches are usually connected through a trailing wire to a computer, although alternatively either a

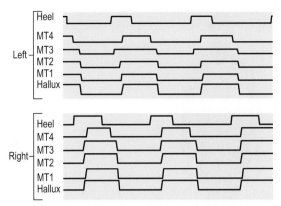

Fig. 4.3 • Output from footswitches under the heel, four metatarsals (MT1 to MT4) and hallux of both feet. The switch is 'on' (i.e. the area is in contact with the ground) when the line is high.

radio transmitter or a portable recording device may be used to collect the data and transfer them to the measuring equipment.

A footswitch is exposed to very high forces, which may cause problems with reliability. This has led to many different designs being tried over the years. A fairly reliable footswitch may be made from two layers of metal mesh, separated by a thin sheet of plastic foam with a hole in it. When pressure is applied, the sheets of mesh contact each other through the hole and complete an electrical circuit. Footswitches are most conveniently used with shoes, although suitably designed ones may be taped directly beneath the foot. Small switches may also be mounted in an insole and worn inside the shoe. In addition to the basic heel and forefoot switches, further switches may be used in other areas of the foot, to give greater detail on the temporal patterns of loading and unloading. In addition to the home-made varieties, a number of companies also manufacture footswitches.

Instrumented walkways

An instrumented walkway is used to measure the timing of foot contact, the position of the foot on the ground, or both. Many different designs have been developed, usually individually built for a single laboratory. The descriptions which follow refer to typical designs, rather than to any particular system.

A conductive walkway is a gait analysis walkway which is covered with an electrically conductive substance, such as sheet metal, metal mesh or conductive rubber. Suitably positioned electrical contacts on the subject's shoes complete an electrical circuit. The conductive walkway is thus a slightly different method of implementing footswitches and provides essentially the same information. Again, the subject usually trails an electrical cable, which connects the foot contacts to a computer. The speed needs to be determined independently, typically by having the body of the subject interrupt the beams of two photoelectric cells, one at each end of the walkway, again connected to the computer. Timing information from the foot contacts is used to calculate the cycle time, and the combination of cycle time and speed may be used to calculate the stride length.

An alternative arrangement is to have the walkway itself contain a large number of switch contacts, which detect the position of the foot, as well as the timing of heel contact and toe off. This has the advantage that no trailing wires are required and the walkway can be used to measure both step lengths and the stride length. A number of commercial systems are available to make this type of measurement, often also providing some information on the magnitude of the forces between the foot and the ground. One such system, which is now in common use, is the 'GAITRite' (Bilney et al., 2003; Menz et al., 2004) (Fig. 4.4).

Camera-based motion analysis

Kinematics is the measurement of movement or, more specifically, the geometrical description of motion, in terms of displacements, velocities and accelerations. Kinematic systems are used in gait analysis to record the position and orientation of the body segments, the angles of the joints, and the corresponding linear and angular velocities and accelerations.

Following the pioneering work of Marey and Muybridge in the 1870s, photography remained the method of choice for the measurement of human movement for about 100 years, until it was replaced by electronic systems. Two basic photographic techniques were used: *cine photography* and *multiple-exposure photography*. Cine photography is achieved by the use of a series of separate photographs, taken in quick succession. Multiple exposure photography has existed in many different forms over the years. It is based on the use of a single photograph, or a strip of film on which a series of images are superimposed,

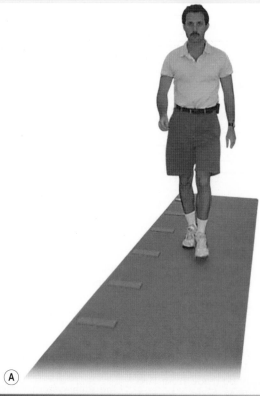

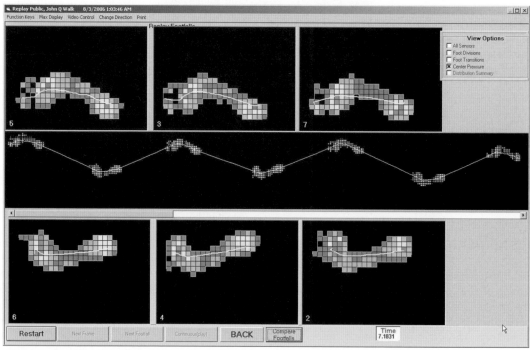

Fig. 4.4 • GAITRite™ system (A) and typical output (B).

sometimes with a horizontal displacement between each image and the next. The 1960s and 1970s saw the development of gait analysis systems based on *optoelectronic techniques*, including television, and these have now superseded photographic methods. The general principles of kinematic measurement are common to all systems and will be discussed before considering particular systems in detail.

General principles

Kinematic measurement may be made in either two dimensions or three. Three-dimensional measurements usually require the use of two or more cameras, although methods have been devised in which a single camera can be used to make limited three-dimensional measurements.

The simplest kinematic measurements are made using a single camera, in an uncalibrated system. Such measurements are fairly inaccurate but they may be useful for some purposes. Without calibration, it is impossible to measure distances accurately and such a system is usually used only to measure joint angles in the sagittal plane. The camera is positioned at right angles to the plane of motion and as far away as possible, to minimise the distortions introduced by perspective. To give a reasonable size image, with a long camera-to-subject distance, a 'telephoto' (long focal length) lens is used. The angles measured from the image are projections of three-dimensional angles onto a two-dimensional plane and any part of the angulation which occurs out of that plane is ignored. Commercial systems of this type are available for measuring joint angles from television images. Such measurements may be subject to yet another form of error, since the horizontal and vertical scales of a television image may be different.

A single-camera system can be used to make approximate measurements of distance, if some form of calibration object is used, such as a grid of known dimensions behind the subject. Measurement accuracy will be lost by any movement towards or away from the camera, but this effect can again be minimised if the camera is a long distance away from the subject, using a telephoto lens. Angulations of the limb segments, either towards or away from the camera, will also interfere with length measurements.

To achieve reasonable accuracy in kinematic measurement, it is necessary to use a calibrated three-dimensional system, which involves making measurements from more than one viewpoint.

A detailed review of the technical aspects of the three-dimensional measurement of human movement was given in four companion papers by Cappozzo et al. (2005), Chiari et al. (2005), Leardini et al. (2005) and Della Croce et al. (2005). Although there are considerable differences in convenience and accuracy between cine film, video recording, television/computer and optoelectronic systems, the data processing for the different types of three-dimensional measurement systems is similar.

Most commercial kinematic systems use a three-dimensional calibration object, which is viewed by all the cameras, either simultaneously or in sequence. Computer software is used to calculate the relationship between the known three-dimensional positions of 'markers' on the calibration object and the two-dimensional positions of those markers in the fields of view of the different cameras. An alternative method of calibration is used by the Codamotion system, whose optoelectronic sensors are in fixed relation to each other, permitting the system to be calibrated in the factory.

When a subject walks in front of the cameras, the calibration process is reversed and three-dimensional positions are calculated for the markers fixed to the subject's limbs, so long as they are visible to at least two cameras. Data are collected at a series of time intervals known as 'frames'. Most systems have an interval between frames of either 20 ms, 16.7 ms or 5 ms, corresponding to data collection frequencies of 50 Hz, 60 Hz or 200 Hz, with some systems now offering frame rates of up to 500 Hz and beyond. When a marker can be seen by only one camera, its three-dimensional position cannot be calculated, although it may be estimated by 'interpolation', using data from earlier and later frames.

All measurement systems, including the kinematic systems to be described, suffer from measurement errors. Measurement accuracy depends to a large extent on the field of view of the cameras, although it also differs somewhat between the different systems. The earlier systems had measurement errors of 2–3 mm in all three dimensions, throughout a volume large enough to cover a complete gait cycle (Whittle, 1982). Recently, design and (especially) calibration improvements have reduced typical errors to less than 1 mm. Some commercial systems claim to provide much higher accuracy than this, but the authors treat such claims with scepticism, particularly when applied to the measurement of moving markers under realistic gait laboratory conditions.

Technical descriptions of kinematic systems use, and sometimes misuse, the terms 'resolution', 'precision' and 'accuracy'. In practical terms, *resolution* means the ability of the system to measure small changes in marker position. *Precision* is a measure of system 'noise', being based on the amount of variability there is between one frame of data and the next. For the majority of users, the most important parameter is *accuracy*, which describes the relationship between where the markers really are and where the system says they are!

Most commercial systems are sufficiently accurate to measure the positions of the limbs and the angles of the joints. However, the calculation of linear or angular velocity requires the mathematical differentiation of the position data, which magnifies any measurement errors. A second differentiation is required to determine acceleration, and a small amount of measurement 'noise' in the original data leads to wildly erratic and often unusable results for acceleration. The usual way of avoiding this problem is to smooth the position data, using a low-pass filter, before differentiation. This achieves the desired object but means that any genuinely high accelerations, such as that at the heelstrike transient, may be lost.

Thus, kinematic systems are good at measuring position but poorer at determining acceleration, because of the problems of differentiating even slightly noisy data. Conversely, accelerometers are good at measuring acceleration but poor at estimating position, because of the problems of integrating data with baseline drift. Really accurate data could be obtained by combining the two methods, using each to correct the other and calculating the velocity from both. Some research studies have been conducted using this combined approach.

As well as the errors inherent in measuring the positions of the markers, further errors are introduced because considerable movement may take place between a skin marker and the underlying bone. A few studies have been performed (e.g. Holden et al., 1997; Reinschmidt et al., 1997) in which steel pins were inserted into the bones of 'volunteers' (usually the investigators themselves) and the positions of skin markers compared with the positions of markers on the pins. The amount of skin movement revealed by such studies is generally somewhat worrying! The amount of error this causes in the final result depends on which parameter is being measured. For example, marker movement has little effect on the sagittal plane knee angle, because it causes only a small relative change in the length of fairly long segments, but it may cause considerable errors in transverse plane measurements or on measurements involving shorter segments, such as in the foot. In some cases, the magnitude of the error is greater than the measurement itself! Skin movement may also introduce errors in the calculation of joint moments and powers. A possibility for the future is to correct for marker movement, by estimating the movement relative to the underlying bone. A further error is introduced when the positions of the joints are estimated from anthropometric measures (e.g. leg length) and the positions of skin markers, particularly where it is possible to place the markers in the wrong position. Even for subjects with normal anatomy, these errors can be substantial; for patients with bony deformity, the errors may be even greater. For these reasons the development of marker sets and anatomical models has been at the forefront of the evolution of gait analysis alongside the ability of new motion analysis systems capable of coping with larger numbers of markers.

Camera-based systems

The use of video to augment visual gait analysis has already been described. Video recording may also be used as the basis for a kinematic system. This has considerable advantages in terms of cost, convenience and speed, although it is not as accurate, due to the poorer resolution of a video image and the sampling frequency compared with data collected from motion analysis cameras. Another considerable advantage, however, is that it is possible to automate the digitisation process using electronic processing of the image, especially if skin markers are used, which show up clearly against the background. A number of commercial systems are available, which can be used either as a two-dimensional system with a single camera, or as a three-dimensional system using two or more cameras. Most video recording systems use conventional television equipment, although high-speed systems are also available.

A number of different camera-based motion capture systems have been developed over the years. Although the systems differ in detail, the following description is typical. Reflective markers are fixed to the subject's limbs, either close to the joint centres or fixed to limb segments in such a way as to identify their positions and orientations. Close to the lens of each camera is an infrared or visible light source (Fig 4.5), which causes the markers to show up as very bright spots (Fig. 4.7).

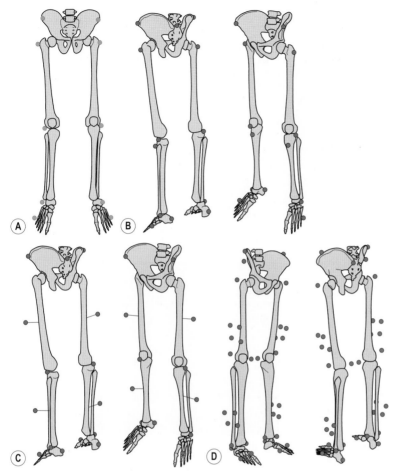

Fig. 4.5 • Common marker sets: (A) simple marker set; (B) Vaughan marker set; (C) Helen Hayes marker set; and (D) Calibrated Anatomical System Technique (CAST).

The markers are usually covered in 'Scotchlite', the material that makes road signs show up brightly when illuminated by car headlights. To avoid 'smearing', which occurs if the marker is moving, only a short exposure time is used. This may be achieved by one or more of the following:

1. Using stroboscopic illumination
2. Using a mechanical shutter on the camera
3. Using a charge-coupled device (CCD) camera, which is only enabled (i.e. activated) for a short interval during each frame.

If two or more cameras are used, much more accurate measurements can be made if they are synchronised. For normal purposes, frame rates of 50 Hz, 60 Hz or 200 Hz are used, although most systems are now able to collect at frame rates up to 500 Hz without loss of pixel resolution. Cameras are either connected via a special interface board, e.g. VICON or 'daisy chained', e.g. Qualisys (Fig. 4.6), both methods allow each frame to be synchronised. Most commercially available systems locate the 'centroid' or geometric centre of each marker within the camera image, but it is typically calculated using the edges of any bright spots in the field of view (Fig. 4.8). Because a large number of edges are used to calculate the position of the centroid, its position can be determined to a greater accuracy than the horizontal and vertical resolution of the image. This is known as making measurements with 'subpixel accuracy'. Marker centroids may also be calculated using the optical density of all the pixels in the image,

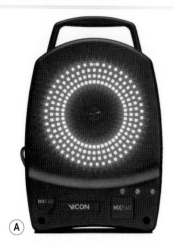
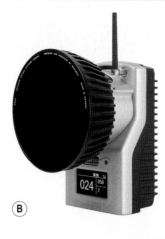

Fig. 4.6 • (A) VICON camera; and (B) Oqus Qualisys camera.

(A)

(B)

rather than just marker edges, again with an improvement in accuracy.

The computer stores the marker centroids from each frame of data for each camera, but initially there is no way to associate a particular marker centroid with a particular physical marker. The process of identifying which marker image is which for each of the cameras, and of following the markers from one frame of data to the next, is known as 'tracking' (Fig. 4.9). The speed and convenience of this process differ considerably from one system to another. In the past this has been the least satisfactory aspect of motion capture systems, however many systems are now capable of real-time marker identification, allowing for much more straightforward and quicker analysis. Whichever method is used the end result of the tracking and three-dimensional reconstruction process is a computer file of three-dimensional marker positions.

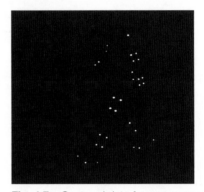

Fig. 4.7 • Captured data from a camera-based system.

Common marker sets

In order to calculate accurate joint kinetics it is essential to locate the centre of rotation of a joint in a repeatable manner through the definition of an anatomical frame. This issue was highlighted by Della Croce et al. (1999), who identified the errors associated with incorrect anatomical frame definition. Therefore the identification and modelling of joint centres has been key to the assessment of joint moments and powers. Joint centres are generally found by using palpable anatomical landmarks to define the medial-lateral axis of the joint. From these anatomical landmarks the centre of rotation is generally calculated in one of two ways: through the use of

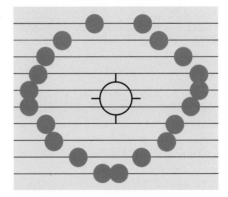

Fig. 4.8 • Location of marker centroid (open circle in centre) from the position on successive television lines of the leading and trailing edges of the marker image (solid circles).

regression equations based on standard radiographic evidence or simply calculated as a percentage offset from the anatomical marker based on some kind of anatomical landmark (Bell et al., 1990; Cappozzo

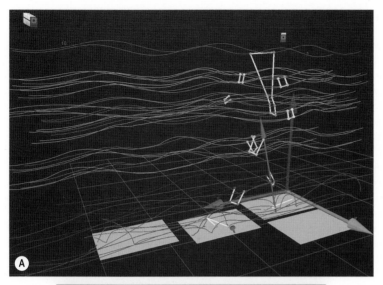

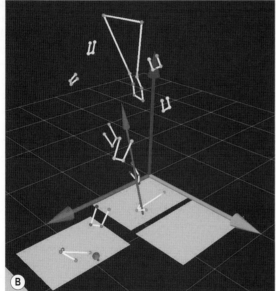

Fig. 4.9A,B • Automatic digitising of a full body Calibrated Anatomical System Technique (CAST) marker set using Qualisys Track Manager.

et al., 1995; Davis et al., 1991; Kadaba et al., 1989). We will now consider several commonly used marker sets which illustrate how improvements have continued to be made.

The simplest marker set involves directly fixing markers on the skin over a bony anatomical landmark close to the centre of rotation of a joint. The position and orientation of the limb segment is then defined by the straight line between the two markers (Fig. 4.5A). This method requires fewer markers

and so theoretically has less interference with the movement pattern, but does not allow the calculation of axial rotation of the body segment. The anatomical landmarks generally used are: head of the fifth metatarsal, lateral malleolus, lateral epicondyle of the femur, greater trochanter and anterior superior iliac spine.

The Vaughan marker set consists of 15 markers on the lower limb and pelvis (Fig. 4.5B). This allows for more detail for the location of the knee joint centre by including a marker in the coronal plane on the tibial tuberosity. The inclusion of the heel marker allows a more appropriate functional reference for the long axis of the foot to be determined between this and the metatarsal heads with the pivot point of the foot determined by the malleoli markers. The inclusion of the sacral marker also allows for a more functional reference for pelvis inclination in the sagittal plane and a meaningful measurement of pelvic tilt. The anatomical landmarks used are: head of the fifth metatarsal, lateral malleolus, heel, tibial tuberosity, lateral femoral epicondyle, greater trochanter, anterior superior iliac spine and sacrum.

The conventional gait model, which is sometimes referred to as the Helen Hayes marker set (Fig. 4.5C), also includes a heel marker and the sacral marker for a more appropriate functional reference for the foot and pelvis. The conventional gait model marker set also includes tibial and femoral wands. Each of these comprises a single marker on a short stick, which is attached to a pad fixed to the segment using tape or bandage. These are not placed on any anatomical position as such and variations on the length of wand and positioning, anterior versus lateral, have been used. The inclusion of these wands allows femoral and tibial rotations to be quantified. The joint markers are placed on anatomical landmarks including: head of the second metatarsal, lateral malleolus, heel, lateral femoral epicondyle, anterior superior iliac spines and either the sacrum or on the posterior superior iliac spines.

The pelvis can be imagined as an equilateral triangle with its front edge formed by the line between the anterior superior iliac spine markers and mid-point of the posterior superior iliac spine markers. The hip joint centre is assumed to be fixed in relation to this triangle at a position estimated using regression equations. The thigh segment can be imagined as another equilateral triangle with its apex between the hip joint centre and the centre of the base at the knee joint axis. This is assumed to pass through the knee in the plane defined by a lateral knee marker, the thigh marker and the hip joint centre. The knee joint centre is defined as lying half the knee width along this axis from the knee marker. The tibia segment is modelled in a similar way to the femur. The foot is defined on the basis of the line between the ankle joint centre and the toe marker. This method does not require the inclusion of joint markers on the medial side and therefore can be potentially susceptible to errors in the estimation of the rotational axis as it uses a medial projection of both the knee and the ankle markers.

The Calibrated Anatomical System Technique (CAST, Fig. 4.5D), was first proposed by Cappozzo et al. (1995) to contribute towards standardising movement description in research labs and clinical centres for the pelvis and lower limb segments. This method involves identifying an anatomical frame for each segment through the identification of anatomical landmarks and segment tracking markers, or marker clusters. Anatomical markers are placed on both the lateral and medial aspects of joints to further improve the estimation of the joint centres. Marker clusters are placed on each body segment. The exact placement of the clusters does not matter, although positioning them on the distal third of the body segment is usual. At least three markers are required to track each segment position and orientation in six degrees of freedom (Cappozzo et al., 2005), however up to nine have been used. The usually accepted number is four or five markers per cluster, allowing for one or two markers to be lost. This is sometimes referred to as marker redundancy, i.e. if you lose a marker during tracking the model will still work. This method determines the position and orientation of each body segment separately, which then allows each joint to be assessed in what is referred to as six degrees of freedom. Six degrees of freedom is best thought of as: three orientations of rotation (i.e. flexion/extension, abduction/adduction, internal/external rotation), and three orientations of translation (i.e. anterior posterior and medial lateral translation, and compression and distraction), although the translational movements are more susceptible to soft tissue movement artefacts.

Active marker systems

Another type of kinematic system uses active markers, typically light-emitting diodes (LEDs), and an array of optoelectronic photo diodes. Among these systems the most common are Codamotion (Fig. 4.10) and Optotrack. Codamotion performs a correlation between the shadow cast on the array by a shadow mask of lines when the LED flashes and a software template of the shadow. This makes use of information from all photodiodes in the array to calculate the 3D marker positions. Optotrak forms a line image of the LED on a CCD Array using a toroidal lens to identify the position of the LED. Typically, these systems use invisible infra-red radiation, but for the sake of clarity, the word 'light' will be used in the following explanation.

In contrast, active markers produce light at a given frequency, so these systems do not require illumination and as such the markers are more easily

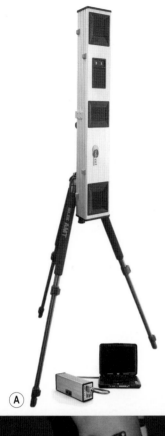

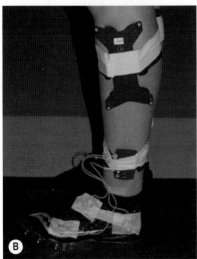

Fig. 4.10 • (A) Codamotion Opto-electronic movement analysis system (Charnwood Dynamics). (B) Codamotion Active LED marker clusters (Charnwood Dynamics).

identified and tracked (Chiari et al., 2005). The most frequently used active markers are those that emit an infra-red signal such as LEDs (Woltring, 1976). LEDs are attached to a body segment in the same way as passive markers, but with the addition of a power source and a control unit for each LED. Active markers can have their own specific frequency which allows them to be automatically detected. This leads to very stable real-time 3D motion tracking as no markers can be misidentified for adjacent markers. Active markers also have the advantage that they can be used outside, as passive marker systems are usually confined to indoors as they are sensitive to in-candescent light and sunlight.

The LEDs are arranged to flash on and off in se-quence, so that only one is illuminated at any instant of time. The photo diodes are thus able to locate each marker in turn, without the need for a 'tracking' pro-cedure to determine which one is which. The penalty for this convenience is the need for the subject to carry a small power supply, with wires running to each of the markers. However Codamotion provide 4-marker clusters (Fig. 4.10) which are synchronized optically and require no wires. Problems may also oc-cur because the photo diodes record not just the light from the LEDs, but any other light which falls on them. This may include stray ambient light, which is fairly easy to eliminate, and also reflections caused by the markers themselves, however in most systems these problems are largely eliminated.

Electrogoniometers and potentiometer devices

An electrogoniometer is a device for making continuous measurements of the angle of a joint. The output of an electrogoniometer is usually plotted as a chart of joint angle against time, as shown in Figure 2.5. However, if measurements have been made from two joints (typ-ically the hip and the knee), the data may be plotted as an *angle-angle diagram*, also known as a 'cyclogram' (Fig. 4.11). This format allows the interaction between the two joints to be plotted on one graph and makes it possible to identify characteristic patterns, although these can sometimes be confusing to interpret.

A rotary potentiometer is a variable resistor of the type used as a radio volume control, in which turning the central spindle produces a change in electrical re-sistance, which can be measured by an external cir-cuit. It can be used to measure the angle of a joint if it is fixed in such a way that the body of the poten-tiometer is attached to one limb segment and the spindle to the other. The electrical output thus depends on the joint position and the device can be calibrated to measure the joint angle in degrees.

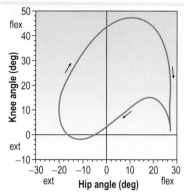

Fig. 4.11 • Angle-angle diagram of the sagittal plane hip angle (horizontal axis) and knee angle (vertical axis). Initial contact is at the lower right. Normal subject; same data as Figure 2.5.

Although any joint motion could be measured by an electrogoniometer, they are most commonly used for the knee and less commonly for the ankle and hip. Fixation is usually achieved by cuffs, which wrap around the limb segment above and below the joint. The position of the potentiometer is adjusted to be as close to the joint axis as possible. A single potentiometer will only make measurements in one axis of the joint, but two or three may be mounted in different planes to make multi-axial measurements (Fig. 4.12). Trailing wires are usually used to connect the potentiometers to the measuring equipment, which is usually a computer. Concern has been expressed about the accuracy of measurement provided by these potentiometer devices, since they are subject to a number of possible types of error, described below.

1. The electrogoniometer is fixed by cuffs around the soft tissues, not to the bones, so that the output of the potentiometer does not exactly relate to the true bone-on-bone movement at the joint.

2. Some designs of electrogoniometer will only give a true measurement of joint motion if the potentiometer axis is aligned to the anatomical axis of the joint. This may not be achievable for three reasons:

   (i) it may be difficult to identify the joint axis, e.g. because of the depth of the hip joint below the surface

   (ii) the joint axis may not be fixed, e.g. the 'polycentric' flexion–extension axis of the knee

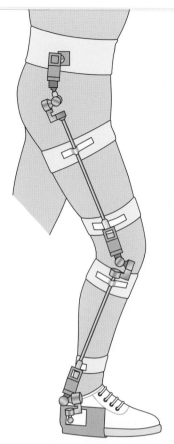

Fig. 4.12 • Subject wearing triaxial goniometers on hip, knee and ankle (adapted from manufacturer's literature (Chattecx Corporation)).

   (iii) the rotation axis may be inaccessible, e.g. the internal–external rotation axis of the knee.

3. A joint may, in theory, move with up to six degrees of freedom – that is, it may have angular motion about three mutually perpendicular axes and linear motion 'translations' in three directions. In practice, the linear motion is usually negligible, particularly at the hip and ankle, and most electrogoniometer systems simply 'lose' any motion which does occur, either through the elasticity of the mounting cuffs or through a sliding or 'parallelogram' mechanical linkage. However, where the electrogoniometer axis does not correspond exactly with the anatomical axis, larger linear motions will occur.

4. The output of the device gives a relative angle rather than an absolute one and it may be difficult to decide what limb angle should be taken as 'zero', particularly in the presence of a fixed deformity.

Because of these problems, electrogoniometers are more popular in a clinical setting, in which great accuracy is not usually needed, than in the scientific laboratory. Chao (1980) addressed some of these problems in a defence of the use of potentiometer-based electrogoniometers in gait analysis.

Flexible strain gauge electrogoniometer

The flexible strain gauge electrogoniometer (Fig. 4.13), manufactured by Biometrics (Cwmfelinfach, Gwent, UK), consists of a flat, thin strip of metal, one end of which is fixed to the limb on each side of the joint being studied. The bending of the metal as the joint moves is measured by strain gauges and their associated electronics. Because of the way in which metal strips respond to bending, the output depends simply on the angle between the two ends, linear motion being ignored. To measure motion in more than one axis, a two-axis goniometer may be used, or two or three separate goniometers may be fixed around the joint, aligned to different planes.

Other electrogoniometers

With the increasing use of camera-based kinematic systems (see above), electrogoniometers are declining in popularity. Other designs which have been used in the past include mercury-in-rubber, in which the electrical resistance of a column of mercury in an elastic tube changes as the tube is stretched across a

joint, and an optical system known as the polarised light goniometer.

Accelerometers

Accelerometers, as their name suggests, measure acceleration. Typically, they contain a small mass, connected to a stiff spring, with some electrical means of measuring the spring deflection when the mass is accelerated. The type of accelerometer used in gait analysis is usually very small, weighing only a few grams. It usually only measures acceleration in one direction, but more than one may be grouped together for two or three dimensional measurements. Solid-state accelerometers, built as integrated circuits, are also available. Because of their small size, they may be of value in gait analysis and also in providing feedback for future systems involving powered artificial limbs and orthoses. Typically, accelerometers have been used for gait analysis in one of two ways: either to measure transient events or to measure the motion of the limbs.

Measurement of transients with accelerometers

Accelerometers are suitable for measuring brief, high-acceleration events, such as the heelstrike transient. Johnson (1990) described the development of an accelerometer system to assess the performance of shock-attenuating footwear, which was made available commercially. The main difficulty with this type of measurement is in obtaining an adequate mechanical linkage between the accelerometer and the skeleton, since slippage occurs in both the skin and the subcutaneous tissues. On a few occasions, experiments have been performed with accelerometers

Fig. 4.13 • Subject wearing flexible goniometers on knee and ankle (adapted from manufacturer's literature (Biometrics)).

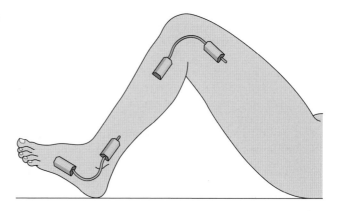

mounted on pins, screwed directly into the bones of volunteers. Reviews of this subject were published by Collins and Whittle (1989) and Whittle (1999).

Measurement of motion with accelerometers

The use of accelerometers for the kinematic analysis of limb motion has been explored by a number of authors, notably Morris (1973). If the acceleration of a limb segment is known, a single mathematical integration will give its velocity and a second integration its position, provided both position and velocity are known at some point during the measurement period. However, these requirements, combined with the 'drift' from which accelerometers often suffer, have prevented them from coming into widespread use for this purpose. If the limb rotates as well as changing its position, which is usually the case, further accelerometers are needed to measure the angular acceleration.

Trunk accelerations have been used to measure the general gait parameters (Zijlstra and Hof, 2003). This is an extension of the principle behind the 'pedometer', often carried by hikers, which counts steps by measuring the vertical accelerations of the trunk.

Gyroscopes, magnetic fields and motion capture suits

It was suggested in the late twentieth century that gyroscopes could be used to measure the orientation of the body segments in space and that 'rate-gyros' could be used to measure angular velocity and acceleration. Gyroscopes were used on an experimental basis in some gait laboratories and the development of very small solid-state devices may make this a useful method of measurement in the future. Nene et al. (1999) used a gyroscope, in combination with several accelerometers, in a study of thigh and shank motion during the swing phase of gait. Several systems were also developed which could detect the position and orientation of a magnetometer sensor, which measures movement relative to magnetic fields. One example was a method for measuring motion of the lumbar spine developed by Pearcy and Hindle (1989), which used a source (transmitter) mounted on the sacrum and a sensor (receiver) over the first lumbar vertebra. Systems are also available in which

the location of ultrasound transmitters, placed on the subject, is detected by an array of microphones.

In the past 10 years considerable advances have been made in motion capture suits, at first in the gaming and animation industries, however these systems are now sensitive and reliable enough to be used in biomechanics and gait analysis. One such system is XSENS MVN motion capture suit (Fig. 4.14). This uses miniature three-dimensional (3D) gyroscopes, accelerometers and magnetometers. These systems require no cameras and do not require markers to be 'seen'. Therefore they can be used indoors and outdoors regardless of lighting conditions. The combination of the three types of sensor allows the tracking of each segment in six degrees of freedom of up to 17 body segments. These systems do sometimes suffer from 'drift' and it is often difficult to obtain a global reference which prevents them being linked with force platforms, however, the relative movement of one body segment about another has been shown to be accurate.

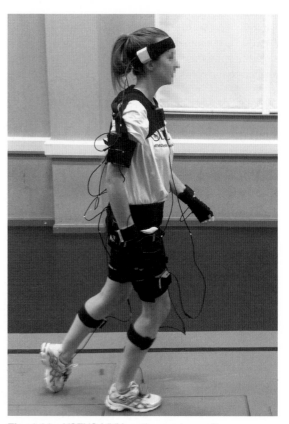

Fig. 4.14 • XSENS MVN motion capture suit.

Measuring force and pressure

Force platforms

The force platform, which is also known as a 'force-plate', is used to measure the ground reaction force as a subject walks across it (Fig. 4.15). Although many specialised types of force platform have been developed over the years, most clinical laboratories use a commercial platform, a 'typical' design being about 100 mm high, with a flat rectangular upper surface measuring 400 mm by 600 mm. To make the upper surface extremely rigid, it is either made of a large piece of metal or of a lightweight honeycomb structure. Within the platform, a number of transducers are used to measure tiny displacements of the upper surface, in all three axes, when force is applied to it. The electrical output of the platform may be provided as either eight channels or six. An eight-channel output consists of:

1. Four vertical signals, from transducers near the corners of the platform
2. Two fore–aft signals from the sides of the platform
3. Two side-to-side signals, from the front and back of the platform.

A six-channel output generally consists of:

1. Three force vector magnitudes
2. Three moments of force, in a coordinate system based on the centre of the platform.

Although it is possible to use the output signal from a force platform directly, for example by displaying it on an oscilloscope, it is much more usual to collect it into a computer, through an analogue-to-digital converter. Neither the eight-channel nor the six-channel force platform output is particularly convenient for

biomechanical calculations and it is usual to convert the data to some other form. Regrettably, no standard has been established for the coordinate systems used for either kinetic or kinematic data.

Ideally, a force platform should be mounted below floor level, the upper surface being flush with the floor. If this is not possible, it is usual to build a slightly raised walkway, to accommodate the thickness of the platform. It is highly undesirable to have the subject step up onto the platform and then down off it again, since such a step could never be regarded as 'normal' walking. Force platforms are very sensitive to building vibrations and many early gait laboratories were built in basements, to reduce this form of interference. In the authors' opinion, this problem has been overemphasised, since although building vibrations can be seen in force platform data, they are negligible when compared with the magnitude of the signals recorded from subjects walking on the platform.

One problem which may be experienced when using force platforms is that of 'aiming'. To obtain good data, the whole of the subject's foot must land on the platform. It is tempting to tell the subject where the platform is and to ask them to make sure that their footstep lands squarely on it. However, this is likely to lead to an artificial gait pattern, as the subject 'aims' for the platform. If at all possible, the platform should be disguised so that it is not noticeably different from the rest of the floor and the subject should not be informed of its presence. This may require a number of walks to be made, with slight adjustments in the starting position, before acceptable data can be obtained.

Where it is required to record from both feet, the relative positioning of two force platforms can be a considerable problem. There is no single arrangement which is satisfactory for all subjects, and some laboratories have designed systems in which one or both platforms can be moved, to suit the gait of individual subjects. Figure 4.16 shows the arrangement used in a number of laboratories, which is a reasonable compromise for studies on adults but is unsatisfactory when the stride length is either very short or very long. For subjects who have a very short stride length, such as children or patients with disorders such as multiple sclerosis, better results may be obtained if the platforms are mounted with their shorter dimensions in the direction of the walk. Alternatively, the direction of the walk may be altered, to cross the platforms diagonally. Despite these strategies, the problem may be insoluble. For example, Gage

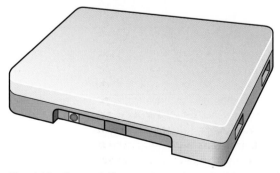

Fig. 4.15 • Force platform (adapted from manufacturer's literature (AMTI)).

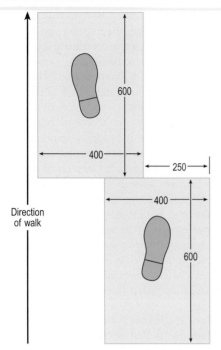

Fig. 4.16 • Typical arrangement of two force platforms for use in studies of adults (dimensions in mm).

Direction of walk

et al. (1984) observed that 'force plate data were discounted because the smaller children frequently stepped on the same platform twice because of their short stride lengths'. Some laboratories improve their chances of obtaining good data by using three or four force platforms.

It is often impossible to get the whole of one foot on one force platform and the whole of the other foot on the other one, without also having unwanted additional steps on one or other platform. To some extent, computer software can be used to 'unscramble' the data when both feet have stepped on one platform but, more commonly, it is necessary to use the data from only one foot at a time.

The usual methods of displaying force platform data are:

1. Individual components, plotted against time (see Fig. 2.20)
2. The 'butterfly diagram' (see Fig. 2.9)
3. The centre of pressure (see Figs 2.21).

In the latter case, if it is required to superimpose a foot outline in the correct position on the plot, it is necessary also to measure the position of the foot on the force platform, for example by using talcum powder.

A number of things have to be borne in mind when interpreting force platform data. Firstly, although the foot is the only part of the body in contact with the platform, the forces which are transmitted by the foot are derived from the mass and inertia of the whole body. The force platform has been described as a 'whole-body accelerometer'; its output gives the acceleration in three-dimensional space of the centre of gravity of the body as a whole, including both the limb that is on the ground and the leg which is swinging through the air. This means that changes in total body inertia may swamp small changes in ground reaction force due to events occurring within the foot. For example, fairly high moments are recorded about the vertical axis during the stance phase of gait (Fig. 4.17). While these may be slightly modified by local events within the foot, they are mainly derived from the acceleration and retardation of the other leg, as it goes through the swing phase. The reaction to the forces responsible for this acceleration and retardation are transmitted to the floor through the stance phase leg and appear in the force platform output, principally as a torque about the vertical axis.

When interpreting force platform data, it is also helpful to remember that force is equivalent to the rate of change of momentum. If two objects of identical mass are dropped onto a force platform from the same height, the one which bounces will produce a higher ground reaction force than one that does not. This may at first seem surprising, until it is

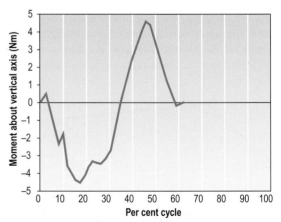

Fig. 4.17 • Moments about the vertical axis at the instantaneous centre of pressure, during the stance phase of gait. Normal subject, right leg. A positive moment occurs when the foot attempts to move clockwise relative to the floor.

realised that the change in momentum is twice as much for the object which bounces as it is for the one that does not. The onset and termination heel-strike transient, shown in Figure 2.23 (page 50), was recorded using a Bertec force platform which has a stiff but lightweight top plate, giving it a high frequency response. When measuring transients, it is important not to pass the data through a low pass filter. If the data are sampled using a computer analogue-to-digital converter, the sampling rate needs to be high enough to record the waveform accurately (the example in Fig. 2.23 used 1000 Hz).

Force platform data by themselves are of limited value in gait analysis. Nevertheless, some laboratories use them empirically, for example by looking for particular patterns in the 'butterfly diagram' (Rose, 1985) or comparing the heights of the different peaks and troughs. Forces, particularly peak vertical force may be looked at for changes over time with an intervention. An example is research on non-steroidal anti-inflammatory drugs used for osteoarthritis to determine if forces increase over time as pain decreases. Some inferences can also be made from the shapes of the curves of the individual force components. For example, there is an association between stance phase flexion of the knee and a dip at mid-stance in the vertical component of force. However, the true value of the force platform is only appreciated when the ground reaction force data are combined with kinematic data. The combination provides a much more complete mechanical description of gait than either by itself and permits the calculation of joint moments and powers.

A number of workers have developed devices which are not force platforms but have the same function. Typically, they consist of a small number of force sensors, which are fixed to the sole of a shoe. As the subject walks, the electrical output gives the ground reaction force and the centre of pressure. Typically only the vertical component of the ground reaction force is measured, although at least one three-axis system has been described. The advantages claimed are:

1. The ability to measure multiple steps
2. No problems with 'aiming'
3. No risk of stepping on the platform with both feet
4. No risk of or missing the platform, either partly or completely.

The disadvantages are the presence of the force sensors beneath the feet, and the associated wiring. Also,

the coordinate system for the force measurements moves with the foot, in contrast to the room-based coordinate system used for kinematic data. This makes it very difficult to combine the two types of data, to perform a full biomechanical analysis.

Force platforms may also be used for balance testing and the measurement of postural sway, which are important in some forms of neurological diagnosis. For a complete analysis of the balance mechanism, however, it is necessary to provide some means whereby both the supporting surface and the visual environment may be moved relative to the subject.

Pressure beneath the foot

The measurement of the pressure beneath the foot is a specialised form of gait analysis, which may be of particular value in conditions in which the pressure may be excessive, such as diabetic neuropathy and rheumatoid arthritis. Lord et al. (1986) reviewed a number of such systems. Foot pressure measurement systems may be either floor mounted or in the form of an insole within the shoe. The SI unit for pressure is the pascal (Pa), which is a pressure of one newton per square metre. The pascal is inconveniently small, and practical measurements are made in kilopascals (kPa) or megapascals (MPa). For conversions between different units of measurement, see Appendix 2.

Lord et al. (1986) pointed out that when making measurements beneath the feet, it is important to distinguish between force and pressure (force per unit area). Some of the measurement systems measure the force (or 'load') over a known area, from which the mean pressure over that area can be calculated. However, the mean pressure may be much lower than the peak pressure within the area if high pressure gradients are present, which are often caused by subcutaneous bony prominences, such as the metatarsal heads.

A pitfall which must be borne in mind when making pressure measurements beneath the feet is that a subject will usually avoid walking on a painful area. Thus, an area of the foot which had previously experienced a high pressure and has become painful may show a low pressure when it is tested. However, this will not happen if the sole of the foot is anaesthetic, as commonly occurs in diabetic neuropathy. In this condition, very high pressures, leading to ulceration, may be recorded.

Typical pressures beneath the foot are 80–100 kPa in standing, 200–500 kPa in walking and up to 1500 kPa in some sporting activities. In diabetic neuropathy, pressures as high as 1000–3000 kPa have been recorded. To put these figures into perspective, the normal systolic blood pressure, measured at the feet in the standing position, is below 33 kPa (250 mmHg); applied pressures which are higher than this will prevent blood from reaching the tissues.

Glass plate examination

Some useful semi-quantitative information on the pressure beneath the foot can be obtained by having the subject stand on, or walk across, a glass plate, which is viewed from below with the aid of a mirror or television camera. It is easy to see which areas of the sole of the foot come into contact with the walking surface and the blanching of the skin gives an idea of the applied pressure. Inspection of both the inside and the outside of a subject's shoe will also provide useful information about the way the foot is used in walking; it is a good idea to ask patients to wear their oldest shoes when they come for an examination, not their newest ones!

Direct pressure mapping systems

A number of low-technology methods of estimating pressure beneath the foot have been described over the years. The Harris or Harris–Beath mat is made of thin rubber, the upper surface of which consists of a pattern of ridges of different heights. Before use, it is coated with printing ink and covered by a sheet of paper, after which the subject is asked to walk across it. The highest ridges compress under relatively light pressures, the lower ones requiring progressively greater pressures, making the transfer of ink to the paper greater in the areas of the highest pressure. This gives a semi-quantitative map of the pressure distribution beneath the foot. Other systems have also been described, in which the subject walks on a pressure-sensitive film, a sheet of aluminium foil or on something like a typist's carbon paper.

Pedobarograph

The pedobarograph uses an elastic mat, laid on top of an edge-lit glass plate. When the subject walks on the mat it is compressed onto the glass, which loses its reflectivity, becoming progressively darker with increasing pressure. This darkening provides the means for quantitative measurement. The underside of the glass plate is usually viewed by a television camera,

the monochrome image being processed to give a 'false-colour' display, in which different colours correspond to different levels of pressure.

Force sensor systems

A number of systems have been described in which the subject walks across an array of force sensors, each of which measures the vertical force beneath a particular area of the foot. Dividing the force by the area of the cell gives the mean pressure beneath the foot in that area. Many different types of force sensor have been used, including resistive and capacitative strain gauges, conductive rubber, piezoelectric materials and a photoelastic optical system. A number of different methods have been used to display the output of such systems, including the attractive presentation shown in Figure 4.18.

In-shoe devices

The problem of measuring the pressure inside the shoe has been tackled in a number of centres. The main difficulties with this type of measurement are the curvature of the surface, a lack of space for the transducers and the need to run large numbers of wires from inside the shoe to the measuring equipment. Nonetheless, a number of commercial systems are now available, which may give clinically useful results. Details of such systems may be found on the internet (see Appendix 3).

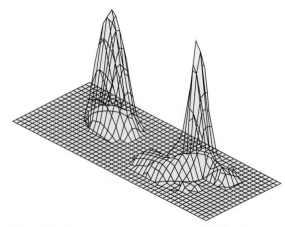

Fig. 4.18 • Pressure beneath a cavus foot on landing from a jump (EM Hennig, 5th Biennial Conference, Canadian Society of Biomechanics, 1988).

Measuring muscle activity

Electromyography

Electromyography (EMG) is the measurement of the electrical activity of a contracting muscle, which is often referred to as the motor unit action potential (MUAP). Since it is a measure of electrical and not mechanical activity, the EMG cannot be used to distinguish between concentric, isometric and eccentric contractions, and the relationship between EMG activity and the force of contraction is far from straightforward. It is particularly good at determining the onset and termination of various muscles contraction during gait (Fig. 4.19). EMG signals have both magnitude and a frequency. The frequency range of the usable EMG signal is between 1 Hz and 500 Hz and the amplitude of the EMG signal varies between 1 µV and 1 mV. The concept of magnitude and frequency can be applied to any signal, but the best way to think about this is the parallel with sound waves. The magnitude of a sound wave is how loud the signal is, and the frequency is the pitch. So with EMG the magnitude of the signal relates to the amount of electric activity during a contraction and the frequency relates to the range of firing rates of all the motor units recorded. One of the most useful textbooks on the EMG is that by Basmajian (1974). The use of the EMG in the biomechanical analysis of movement was reviewed by Kleissen et al. (1998).

The EMG signal may be displayed in a number of ways. Clinical EMG biofeedback devices may display the magnitude of the signal by how many lights can be illuminated with a contraction. However for more scientific study the EMG signal is either displayed as a continuous line which oscillates up and down (Fig. 4.19A), or as a signal power to frequency plot (Fig. 4.19B). The three methods of recording the EMG are by means of surface, fine wire and needle electrodes. In gait analysis, EMG is usually measured with the subject walking, as opposed to the semi-static EMG measurements that are often made for neurological diagnosis.

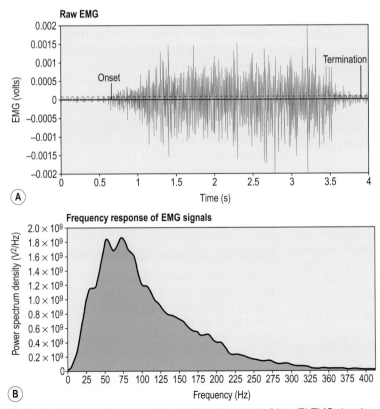

Fig. 4.19 • A) Timing of onset and termination of a muscle firing. (B) EMG signal power to frequency plot.

Surface electrodes

Surface EMG is by far the most widely used method for gait analysis. Surface electrodes are fixed to the skin over the muscle, the EMG being recorded as the voltage difference between two electrodes. It is usually necessary also to have a grounding electrode, either nearby or elsewhere on the body. Since the muscle action potential reaches the electrodes through the intervening layers of fascia, fat and skin, the voltage of the signal is relatively small and it is usually amplified close to the electrodes, using a very small pre-amplifier. The EMG signal picked up by surface electrodes is the sum of the muscle action potentials from many motor units within the most superficial muscle or muscles. Most of the signal comes from within 25 mm of the skin surface, so this type of recording is not suitable for deep muscles such as the iliopsoas. When targeting the EMG of a particular muscle we sometimes pick up activity from adjacent muscles, this is referred to as 'crosstalk'. Therefore it is sometimes safest to regard the signal from surface electrodes as being derived from muscle groups, rather than from individual muscles, although Õunpuu et al. (1997) showed that surface electrodes could satisfactorily distinguish between the three superficial muscle bellies of the quadriceps in children. There is often a change in the electrical baseline as the subject moves ('movement artefact') and there may also be electromagnetic interference, for example from nearby electrical equipment. The authors would recommend studying the wealth of information in the SENIAM guidelines (www.seniam.org) and also on the DelSys website (www.delsys.com).

Fine wire electrodes

Fine wire electrodes are introduced directly into a muscle, using a hypodermic needle which is then withdrawn, leaving the wires in place. They can be quite uncomfortable or even painful. The wire is insulated, except for a few millimetres at the tip. The EMG signal may be recorded in three different ways:

1. Between a pair of wires inserted using a single needle
2. Between two fine wires, inserted separately
3. Between a single fine wire and a ground electrode.

The voltage recorded within the muscle is generally higher than that from surface electrodes, particularly if separate wires are used, and there is less interference from movement and from electromagnetic fields. The signal is derived from a fairly small region

of a single muscle, generally from a few motor units only, a fact which must be taken into account when interpreting the data. Because it is an uncomfortable and invasive technique, fine-wire EMG is usually only performed on selected muscles, in patients in whom it is likely to be particularly useful.

Needle electrodes

Needle electrodes are generally more appropriate to physiological research than to gait analysis. A hypodermic needle is used, which contains an insulated central conductor. This records the EMG signal from a very local area within the muscle into which it is inserted, usually only a single motor unit.

Signal processing of EMG signals

Raw EMG

EMG signals are low voltage, and the signal can be hidden by other electrical noise. Therefore EMG signals have to be amplified to reduce the effect of this noise, typically between 1000 and 10 000 times to give a measurable signal. To decrease electrical interference the amplifiers can be positioned close to the electrodes, which reduces the length of wire that can pick up interference.

Often the EMG signal will oscillate on either side of a floating reference, this is referred to as low voltage offset, or bias. The way to remove bias is to find the mean value of the entire signal and then subtract this from the original signal, therefore pulling the data to a 'zeroed' position. The threshold of the signal can then be set to give information as to whether the muscle is firing or not. This gives an on/off measurement of whether the muscle is active or not, or muscle activity onset and termination.

Rectified, enveloped and integrated EMG

Rectification is required because the raw EMG signal (when the low voltage offset has been removed) oscillates positive and negative either side of the zero line, therefore if we were to try to find the mean value we would end up with zero. Rectification takes the entire signal and makes all the negative values in the signal positive. This can be achieved by first squaring the signal and then taking the square root. This is sometimes preferred when determining the threshold for the onset or termination of muscle contraction (Fig. 4.20A).

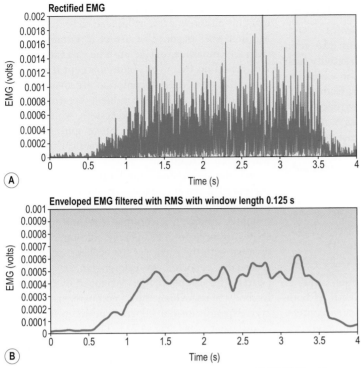

Fig. 4.20 • (A) Rectified EMG. (B) Root mean square (RMS) EMG with a 0.125 s window length.

Enveloped EMG is a common method of showing the level of muscle activity which involves 'filtering' or 'processing' the EMG signal. A low pass filter is used which lets the lower frequencies through while stopping the higher frequencies. The practical upshot of this is a smoothing effect similar to that used in movement analysis. There is much debate as to how much this should be filtered; typical amounts of filtering used in the literature vary between 6 Hz and 25 Hz cut-off frequencies for a low pass filter. Another method of filtering is using the root mean square. The root mean square is calculated using a moving window and the calculation consists of three steps:

1. Squaring each data point in the signal
2. Determining an average value over a specified window length e.g. 0.125 seconds
3. Taking the square root (Fig. 4.20B).

Integrated EMG (iEMG) refers to the area under the full rectified EMG trace. This has been used as an indicator of work done by the muscle. From this the amount of 'relative' work done by a muscle group during push off during walking could be found if the events at the start and end of the push off were identified. Therefore iEMG would give us a single value for this period.

Limitations of EMG

The main problem with the use of any form of EMG is that it is at best only a semi-quantitative technique and gives little indication of the strength of contraction of individual muscles. Many attempts have been made over the years to make it more quantitative, with only limited success. The EMG signal is generally processed to provide a visible indication of muscle activity.

Despite its limitations, the information provided by EMG on the timing of muscle activation can be of considerable value in gait assessment. For example, one form of treatment in cerebral palsy is to transfer the tendon of a muscle to a different position, thereby altering the action of the muscle. When contemplating this type of surgery, it is essential to use EMG first, to make sure that the timing of muscular contraction is appropriate for its new role. It is also possible to determine any relative changes in activity due to immediate treatment, e.g. the use of orthoses, taping and bracing.

Measuring energy expenditure

The most accurate way of measuring the total amount of energy used in performing an activity such as walking is 'whole-body calorimetry', in which the subject is kept in an insulated chamber, from which the heat output of the body can be measured. This is, of course, quite impractical, except as a research technique. The most usual way of estimating energy expenditure is based on measuring the body's oxygen consumption. There are also less direct methods, using either mechanical calculations or the measurement of heart rate.

Oxygen consumption

The measurement of oxygen consumption requires an analysis of the subject's exhaled breath. If both the volume of exhaled air and its oxygen content are measured, the amount of oxygen consumed in a given time can be calculated. The amount of carbon dioxide produced can also be measured and the ratio of the carbon dioxide produced to the oxygen consumed (the 'respiratory quotient') provides information on the type of metabolism that is taking place (aerobic or anaerobic). Except under abnormal environmental conditions, it is not necessary to measure either the oxygen or the carbon dioxide in the inspired air, since these are almost constant.

The classic method of measuring oxygen consumption and carbon dioxide production is to fit the subject with a nose clip and mouthpiece and to collect the whole of the expired air in a large plastic or rubberised canvas 'Douglas bag' or a meteorological balloon. If the subject is walking, some means of following them around with the bag is needed. A small sample of the gas in the bag is then analysed, after which the volume of exhalate in the bag is measured. After correcting for temperature, air pressure and humidity, a very accurate estimate of oxygen consumption can be obtained. However, collecting the expirate in this way is uncomfortable for the subject and the technique is quite unsuitable for some patients.

A less cumbersome, though potentially slightly less accurate method again involves a nose clip and mouthpiece, but uses a portable system which performs continuous gas sampling and volume measurement, so that it is not necessary to collect the whole of the expirate. Either form of gas collection can be achieved using a facemask, rather than a

mouthpiece and nose clip, although it may be very difficult either to prevent leakage or to detect leakage if it does occur. The use of a portable system with a facemask is routine in some gait analysis centres, who find that even children accept it well. Occasionally, studies of locomotion are made using a spirometer, in which the subject breathes in and out of an oxygen-filled closed system, which absorbs the exhaled carbon dioxide. Since spirometers are not usually portable, they are practical only when walking on a treadmill.

Whichever method is used this information can be presented in one of two ways, the energy expenditure per unit time and the energy expenditure per unit distance. Energy expenditure per unit time (E_w) shows an increase in the energy consumed by an individual with the square of the walking speed, which is usually reported as calorie/min or joules/sec (watt). This can be further developed by controlling for body mass, which allows comparison of the energy expenditure per kilogram between individuals of different mass (Fig. 4.21). The measurement of energy per unit distance walked (E_m) provides a quantitative measure of energy economy. Figure 4.22 shows how the energy expenditure per metre walked varies with walking speed. When this value is at a minimum the individual is walking at their most efficient speed. Therefore we can determine that the most efficient walking speed is 1.33 m/s, 80 m/min, 4.7 km/h or 2.9 miles an hour, for normal able-bodied walking. Any increase or decrease in walking speed will cause an increase in the energy expenditure per metre walked and a reduction in efficiency (Corcoran and Brengelmann, 1970; Ralston, 1958). In this way the most efficient walking speed can be found for a particular individual and allows a useful comparison when studying pathological gait.

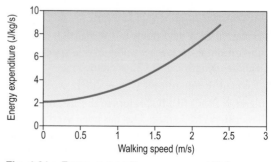

Fig. 4.21 • Energy expenditure per second (E_w) versus walking speed.

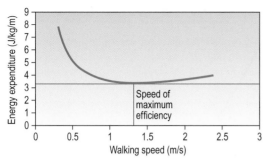

Fig. 4.22 • Energy expenditure per metre (E_m) versus walking speed.

Heart rate monitoring

Rose (1983) stated that heart rate monitoring is a good substitute for the measurement of oxygen uptake, since a number of studies over the years have shown that there is a surprisingly close relationship between the two. Heart rate monitoring is certainly much easier to perform and there are a number of systems available, often based on detecting the pulsatile flow in the capillaries, for example in the finger. Another method of recording heart rate is to detect the electrocardiogram, using electrodes mounted on the chest. As a general rule, the energy consumption is related to the difference in heart rate between the resting condition and that measured during the exercise. Rather than attempting to relate the change in heart rate directly to energy consumption, some investigators use the 'physiological cost index' (PCI), which is said to be less sensitive to differences between individuals (Steven et al., 1983). It is calculated as follows:

$$PCI = (\text{heart rate walking} - \text{heart rate resting})/\text{speed}$$

The calculation must be made using consistent units, with the heart rate in beats per minute and the speed in metres per minute, or the heart rate in beats per second and the speed in metres per second. The measurement unit for the PCI is net beats per metre. Since the heart rate tends to be somewhat variable, small changes in PCI may not be significant; however, PCI gives a comparable pattern to the energy expenditure per metre (E_m).

Mechanical calculations of energy expenditure

It was pointed out in Chapter 1 that the expenditure of metabolic energy does not result in the production of an equivalent amount of mechanical work. Indeed, in eccentric muscular activity, metabolic energy is used to absorb, rather than to generate, mechanical energy. Even when muscular contraction is used to do positive work, the efficiency of conversion is relatively low, as well as being variable and difficult to estimate. For these reasons, it is generally unsatisfactory to use mechanical calculations to estimate the total metabolic energy consumed in a complicated activity such as walking. Nonetheless, this method of estimating energy expenditure is used in some laboratories (Gage et al., 1984) and is known as the 'estimated external work of walking' (EEWW). Calculations of this type are more reliable for activities where the relationship between the muscular contraction and the mechanical output is extremely simple, such as in the concentric contraction of a single muscle.

Even though mechanical calculations are generally unsatisfactory for the estimation of the total energy consumption of the body, the measurement of the energy generation and transfer at individual joints may be of great value in gait analysis. Results of such measurements were given in Chapters 2 and 3. They may be made using combined kinetic/kinematic systems.

Combined kinetic/kinematic systems

When a kinematic system is combined with a force platform (which is a kinetic system), the capability of the combined system is greater than that of the sum of its component parts. The reason for this is that if the relationship is known between the limb segments and the ground reaction force vector, it is possible to perform 'inverse dynamic' calculations, in which the limb is treated as a mechanical system. While not all commercial systems provide the necessary software to make these calculations, there exists the potential to calculate the moments of force and the power generated or absorbed at all the major joints of the lower limb. Such calculations require knowledge of the masses and moments of inertia of the limb segments and the location of their centres of gravity. Direct measurements of these are clearly impossible, but published data, modified to suit the subject's anthropometry, give an acceptable approximation. It is common practice in such calculations to regard the foot as a single rigid object, although this

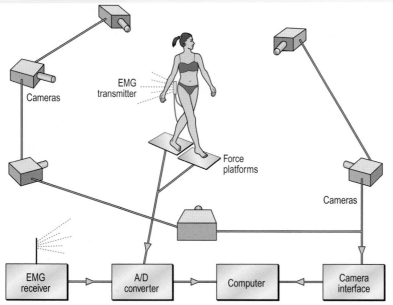

EMG transmitter

Cameras

EMG receiver

A/D converter

Computer

Camera interface

Force platforms

Cameras

Fig. 4.23 • The gait analysis equipment used in the author's laboratory, with a six camera kinematic system, two force platforms and an EMG telemetry system.

simplification undoubtedly causes errors in calculating the ankle power.

A fully equipped clinical gait laboratory can be expected to possess, as a minimum, a combined kinetic/kinematic system, with ambulatory EMG (Fig. 4.23), as well as recording video. Equipment may also be available for measuring oxygen uptake or pressure beneath the feet. If the laboratory is also used for research, then further facilities and equipment may also be present.

One of the big problems with kinetic/kinematic systems is that they provide such a wealth of data that it may be very difficult to distinguish between those observations which are important and those which are not. Recent studies have used a number of mathematical, statistical and computational tech-

niques in an attempt to address this problem (Chau, 2001a,b), some examples being multivariate analysis, principal component analysis, neural networks and the charmingly named 'fuzzy systems'. It may be anticipated that in the future 'expert systems' will be available to draw the attention of clinicians to those aspects of a patient's gait most in need of attention. Another way of coping with this huge quantity of data is to reduce many different measurements to a single index. An example of this is the 'normalcy index' suggested by Schutte et al. (2000) as a method of quantifying a patient's disability and providing an outcome measure to gauge their response to treatment, which Romei et al. (2004) found to be 'clinically applicable, reliable and easy to use'. This will be considered in more detail in Chapter 5.

References

Basmajian, J.V., 1974. Muscles Alive: Their Functions Revealed by Electromyography. Lippincott Williams & Wilkins, Baltimore, MD.

Bell, A., Pederson, D., Brand, R., 1990. A comparison of the accuracy of several hip centre location predication methods. J. Biomech. 23 (6), 617–621.

Bilney, B., Morris, M., Webster, K., 2003. Concurrent related validity of the GAITRite walkway system for quantification of the spatial and temporal parameters of gait. Gait Posture 17, 68–74.

Brandstater, M.E., de Bruin, H., Gowland, C., et al., 1983. Hemiplegic gait: analysis of temporal variables.

Arch. Phys. Med. Rehabil. 64, 583–587.

Cappozzo, A., Catani, F., Croce, U.D., Leardini, A., 1995. Position and orientation in space of bones during movement: anatomical frame definition and determination. Clin. Biomech. (Bristol, Avon) 10 (4), 171–178.

Cappozzo, A., Della Croce, U., Leardini, A., et al., 2005. Human movement analysis using stereophotogrammetry. Part 1: Theoretical background. Gait Posture 21, 186–196.

Chao, E.Y.S., 1980. Justification of triaxial goniometer for the measurement of joint rotation. J. Biomech. 13, 989–1006.

Chau, T., 2001a. A review of analytical techniques for gait data. Part 1: fuzzy, statistical and fractal methods. Gait Posture 13, 49–66.

Chau, T., 2001b. A review of analytical techniques for gait data. Part 2: neural network and wavelet methods. Gait Posture 13, 102–120.

Chiari, L., Della Croce, U., Leardini, A., et al., 2005. Human movement analysis using stereophotogrammetry. Part 2: Instrumental errors. Gait Posture 21, 197–211.

Collins, J.J., Whittle, M.W., 1989. Impulsive forces during walking and their clinical implications. Clin. Biomech. (Bristol, Avon) 4, 179–187.

Corcoran, B., 1970. Oxygen uptake in normal and handicapped subjects, in relation to speed of walking beside velocity controlled cart. Arch. Phys. Med. Rehabil. 51, 78–87.

Davis, R., Ounpuu, S., Tyburski, D., Gage, J., 1991. A gait data collection and reduction technique. Hum. Mov. Sci. 10, 575–587.

Della Croce, U., Cappozzo, A., Kerrigan, D.C., 1999. Pelvis and lower limb anatomical landmark calibration precision and its propagation to bone geometry and joint angles. Med. Biol. Eng. Comput. 37 (2), 155–161.

Della Croce, U., Leardini, A., Chiari, L., et al., 2005. Human movement analysis using stereophotogrammetry. Part 4: Assessment of anatomical landmark misplacement and its effects on joint kinematics. Gait Posture 21, 226–237.

Gage, J.R., Fabian, D., Hicks, R., et al., 1984. Pre- and postoperative gait analysis in patients with spastic diplegia: a preliminary report. J. Pediatr. Orthop. 4, 715–725.

Gerny, K., 1983. A clinical method of quantitative gait analysis. Phys. Ther. 63, 1125–1126.

Hillman, S.J., Hazlewood, M.E., Loudon, I.R., et al., 1998. Can transverse plane rotations be estimated from video tape gait analysis? Gait Posture 8, 87–90.

Holden, J.P., Orsini, J.A., Siegel, K.L., et al., 1997. Surface movement errors in shank kinematics and knee kinetics during gait. Gait Posture 5, 217–227.

Johnson, G.R., 1990. Measurement of shock acceleration during walking and running using the shock meter. Clin. Biomech. (Bristol, Avon) 5, 47–50.

Kadaba, M.P., Ramakrishnan, H.K., Wootten, M.E., Gainey, J., Gorton, G., Cochran, G.V., 1989. Repeatability of kinematic, kinetic, and electromyographic data in normal adult gait. J. Orthop. Res. 7 (6), 849–860.

Kleissen, R.F.M., Buurke, J.H., Harlaar, J., et al., 1998. Electromyography in the biomechanical analysis of human movement and its clinical application. Gait Posture 8, 143–158.

Krebs, D.E., Edelstein, J.E., Fishman, S., 1985. Reliability of observational kinematic gait analysis. Phys. Ther. 65, 1027–1033.

Leardini, A., Chiari, L., Della Croce, U., et al., 2005. Human movement analysis using stereophotogrammetry. Part 3: Soft tissue artifact assessment and compensation. Gait Posture 21, 212–225.

Lord, M., Reynolds, D.P., Hughes, J.R., 1986. Foot pressure measurement: a review of clinical findings. J. Biomed. Eng. 8, 283–294.

Menz, H.B., Latt, M.D., Tiedemann, A., et al., 2004. Reliability of the GAITRite walkway system for the quantification of temporo-spatial parameters of gait in young and older people. Gait Posture 20, 20–25.

Morris, J.R.W., 1973. Accelerometry – a technique for the measurement of human body movements. J. Biomech. 6, 729–736.

Nene, A., Mayagoitia, R., Veltink, P., 1999. Assessment of rectus femoris function during initial swing phase. Gait Posture 9, 1–9.

Õunpuu, S., DeLuca, P.A., Bell, K.J., et al., 1997. Using surface electrodes for the evaluation of the rectus femoris, vastus medialis and vastus lateralis in children with cerebral palsy. Gait Posture 5, 211–216.

Pearcy, M.J., Hindle, R.J., 1989. New methods for the non-invasive three-dimensional measurement of human back movement. Clin. Biomech. (Bristol, Avon) 4, 73–79.

Ralston, H.J., 1958. Energy speed relation and optimal speed during level walking. Int. Z. Angew. Physiol. 17, 277.

Rafferty, D., Bell, F., 1995. Gait analysis – a semiautomated approach. Gait Posture 3 (3), 184.

Reinschmidt, C., van den Bogert, A.J., Lundberg, A., et al., 1997. Tibiofemoral and tibiocalcaneal motion during walking: external vs. skeletal markers. Gait Posture 6, 98–109.

Robinson, J.L., Smidt, G.L., 1981. Quantitative gait evaluation in the clinic. Phys. Ther. 61, 351–353.

Romei, M., Galli, M., Motta, F., et al., 2004. Use of the normalcy index for the evaluation of gait pathology. Gait Posture 19, 85–90.

Rose, G.K., 1983. Clinical gait assessment: a personal view. J. Med. Eng. Technol. 7, 273–279.

Rose, G.K., 1985. Use of ORLAU-Pedotti diagrams in clinical gait assessment. In: Whittle, M., Harris, D. (Eds.), Biomechanical Measurement in Orthopaedic Practice. Clarendon Press, Oxford, pp. 205–210.

Saleh, M., Murdoch, G., 1985. In defence of gait analysis. J. Bone Joint Surg. Br. 67, 237–241.

Schutte, L.M., Narayanan, U., Stout, J.L., et al., 2000. An index for quantifying deviations from normal gait. Gait Posture 11, 25–31.

Steven, M.M., Capell, H.A., Sturrock, R.D., et al., 1983. The physiological cost of gait (PCG): a new technique for evaluating nonsteroidal antiinflammatory drugs in rheumatoid arthritis. Br. J. Rheumatol. 22, 141–145.

Whittle, M.W., 1982. Calibration and performance of a three-dimensional television system for kinematic analysis. J. Biomech. 15, 185–196.

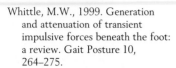

Whittle, M.W., 1999. Generation and attenuation of transient impulsive forces beneath the foot: a review. Gait Posture 10, 264–275.

Whittle, M.W., Levine, D.F., 1997. Measurement of lumbar lordosis as a component of clinical gait analysis. Gait Posture 5, 101–107.

Woltring, H.J., 1976. Calibration and measurement in 3-dimensional monitoring of human motion by optoelectronic means. II. Experimental results and discussion. Biotelemetry 3 (2), 65–97.

Zijlstra, W., Hof, A.L., 2003. Assessment of spatio-temporal gait parameters from trunk accelerations during human walking. Gait Posture 18, 1–10.

Zijlstra, W., Rutgers, A.W.F., Hof, A.L., et al., 1995. Voluntary and involuntary adaptation of walking to temporal and spatial constraints. Gait Posture 3, 13–18.

Further reading

Bilney, B., Morris, M., Webster, K., 2003. Concurrent related validity of the GAITRite walkway system for quantification of the spatial and temporal parameters of gait. Gait Posture 17, 68–74.

Crosbie, J., Vachalathiti, R., Smith, R., 1997. Patterns of spinal motion during walking. Gait Posture 5, 6–12.

Klenerman, L., Dobbs, R.J., Weller, C., et al., 1988. Bringing gait analysis out of the laboratory and into the clinic. Age Ageing 17, 397–400.

Law, H.T., 1987. Microcomputer-based, low cost method for measurement of spatial and temporal parameters of gait. J. Biomed. Eng. 9, 115–120.

Law, H.T., Minns, R.A., 1989. Measurement of the spatial and temporal parameters of gait. Physiotherapy 75, 81–84.

New York University, 1986. Lower Limb Orthotics. New York University Postgraduate Medical School, New York, NY.

Applications of gait analysis

5

Michael Whittle   David Levine   Jim Richards   Gabor Barton

The aim of this chapter is to provide a broad overview of some of the ways in which gait analysis is used, particularly in a clinical setting. It is not intended to transform the reader into an expert on the subject. Anyone planning to use gait analysis in clinical decision making should read all the texts listed at the end of this chapter, attend courses and training on the interpretation of gait analysis data, and if possible spend some time studying or working in a clinical gait laboratory. There are several national and international societies that specialise in such courses and training, such as the European Society of Movement Analysis for Adults and Children (ESMAC), the Gait and Clinical Movement Analysis Society (GCMAS) and the Clinical Movement Analysis Society (CMAS).

The applications of gait analysis are conveniently divided into two main categories: *clinical gait assessment* and *gait research*. Clinical gait assessment has the aim of helping individual patients directly, whereas gait research aims to improve our understanding of gait, either as an end in itself or in order to improve medical diagnosis or treatment in the future. There is obviously some overlap, in that many people performing clinical gait assessment use it as the basis for research studies. Indeed, this is the way that most progress in the use of clinical gait assessment is made.

Davis (1988) pointed out that there are considerable differences between the technical requirements for clinical gait assessment and those for gait research. For example, an intrusive measurement system and a cluttered laboratory environment might not worry a fit adult, who is acting as an experimental subject, but could cause significant changes in the gait of a child with cerebral palsy. In gait research, it might be acceptable to spend a whole day preparing the subject, making the measurements and processing the data, whereas in the clinical setting patients often tire easily and the results are usually needed as quickly as possible. The requirements for accuracy are generally not as great in the clinical setting as they are in the research laboratory, so long as the measurement errors are not large enough to cause a misinterpretation of the clinical condition. However, it is essential that those interpreting the data appreciate the possible magnitude of any such errors. Finally, the system must be able to cope with a wide variety of pathological gaits. It is much easier to make measurements on normal subjects than on those whose gait is very abnormal, which may explain why the literature of the subject is dominated by studies of normal individuals! A final and important point is that there is no value in using a complicated and expensive measurement system, unless it provides information which is useful and which cannot be obtained in an easier way.

Gait research may be divided into clinical and fundamental research, the former concentrating on disease processes and methods of treatment, the latter on methods of measurement and the advancement of knowledge in biomechanics, human performance and physiology.

Clinical gait assessment

Clinical gait assessment seeks to describe, on a particular occasion, the way in which a person walks. This may be all that is required, if the aim is simply to document their current status. Alternatively, it may be just one step in a continuing process, such as the planning of treatment or the monitoring of progress over a period of time.

Rose (1983) made a distinction between gait analysis and gait assessment. He regarded gait analysis as 'data gathering' and gait assessment as 'the integration of this information with that from other sources for the purposes of clinical decision making'. This usage of the term 'analysis' differs from that in more technical fields, in which it means 'the processing of data to derive new information'. However, Rose's use of the term is helpful, because it points out that gait assessment is simply one form of clinical assessment. Medical students are taught that clinical assessment is based on three components: history, physical examination and special investigations. In this context, gait analysis is simply a special investigation, the results of which will augment other investigations, such as X-ray reports and blood biochemistry, to provide a full clinical picture. The term 'gait evaluation' is sometimes used instead of gait analysis.

The simplest form of gait assessment is practised every day in physician offices, physiotherapy and rehabilitation clinics, orthotic and prosthetic clinics, sports centres, and many other settings throughout the world. Every time a clinician watches a client or patient walk up and down a room, they are performing an assessment of the patient's gait. However, such assessment is often unsystematic and the most that can be hoped for is to obtain a general impression of how well the patient walks, and perhaps some idea of one or two of the main problems. This could be termed an 'informal' gait assessment. To perform a 'formal' gait assessment requires a careful examination of the gait, using a systematic approach, if possible, augmented by objective measurements. Such a gait assessment will usually produce a written report and the discipline involved in preparing such a report is likely to result in a much more carefully conducted assessment.

The gait analysis techniques which are used in clinical gait assessment vary enormously, with the nature of the clinical condition, the skills and facilities available in the individual clinic or laboratory and the purpose for which the assessment is being conducted. In general, however, clinical gait assessment is performed for one of three possible reasons: it may form the basis of clinical decision making, it may help with the diagnosis of an abnormal gait, or it may be used to document a patient's condition. These will be considered in turn.

Clinical decision making

Both Rose (1983) and Gage (1983) suggested that clinical decision making in cases of gait abnormality should involve three clear stages.

1. Gait assessment: this starts with a full clinical history, both from the patient and from any others involved, such as doctors, therapists or family members. Where a patient has previously had surgery, details of this should be obtained, if possible from the operative notes. History taking is followed by a physical examination, with particular emphasis on the neuromusculoskeletal system. In many laboratories, physical examinations are performed by both a doctor and a physiotherapist. Finally, a formal gait analysis is carried out.

2. Hypothesis formation: the next stage is the development of a hypothesis regarding the cause or causes of the observed abnormalities. This hypothesis is often informed by the specific questions raised by the referring doctor. Time needs to be set aside to review the data, and consultation between colleagues, particularly those from different disciplines, is extremely valuable. Indeed, almost all of those using gait assessment as a clinical decision-making tool stress the value of this 'team approach'. In forming a hypothesis as to the fundamental problem in a patient with a gait disorder, Rose (1983) emphasised that the patient's gait pattern is not entirely the direct result of the pathology, but is the net result of the original problem and the patient's ability to compensate for it. He observed that the worse the underlying problem, the easier it is to form a hypothesis, since the patient is less able to compensate.

3. Hypothesis testing: this stage is sometimes omitted, when there is little doubt as to the cause of the abnormalities observed. However, where some doubt does exist, the hypothesis can be tested in two different ways – either by using a different method of measurement or by attempting in some way to modify the gait. Some laboratories routinely use a fairly complete 'standard protocol', including video recording, kinematic measurement, force platform measurements and surface electromyography (EMG). They will then add other measurements, such as fine wire EMG, where this is necessary to test a hypothesis. Other clinicians start the gait analysis using a simple method, such as video recording, and only add other techniques, such as EMG or the use of a force platform, where they would clearly be helpful. Rose (1983) opposed the use of a standard protocol for all patients, since some of the procedures turn out to be unnecessary and there is a risk of ending up with 'an exhausted subject in pain'. The other method of testing a hypothesis is to re-examine the gait after attempting some form of modification, typically by the application of an orthosis to limit joint motion, a medication such as botulinum toxin to decrease spasticity, or by anaesthetising a muscle. The ultimate form of gait modification is the surgical operation, with retesting following recovery. However, this is a rather drastic form of 'hypothesis testing', which can be used only where there is a good reason to suppose that the operation will lead to a definite improvement.

Different types of gait analysis data may be useful for different aspects of the gait assessment. Information on foot timing may be useful to identify asymmetries and may indicate problems with balance, stability, pain etc. The general gait parameters give a guide to the degree of disability and may be used to monitor progress or deterioration with the passage of time. The kinematics of limb motion describe abnormal movements, but do not identify the 'guilty' muscles.

The most useful measures are probably the joint moments and joint powers, particularly if this information is supplemented by EMG data. Hemiparetic patients may show greater differences between the two sides in muscle power output than in any of the other measurable parameters, including EMG. Winter (1985) stressed the need to work backwards from the observed gait abnormalities to the underlying causes in terms of the 'guilty' motor patterns, using both the EMG and the moments about the hip, knee and ankle joints. He offered a method of charting gait abnormalities and a table giving the common gait disorders, their possible causes and the type of evidence which would confirm or refute them (Table 5.1). Although the next step, that of treatment, was not considered in detail, he suggested that once an accurate 'diagnosis' had been made, the therapist would be challenged to 'alter or optimise the abnormal motor patterns' which requires the understanding of the biomechanical cause–effect relationships necessary to improve gait.

Many others working in the field of clinical gait assessment have noted the difficulty of deducing the underlying cause from the observed gait abnormalities, because of the compensations which take place. A number of attempts have been made to simplify this process, by using a systematic approach. Computer-based expert systems are very suitable for this type of application and a number of such systems have been developed for clinical gait assessment. Since gait patterns are seldom clear-cut, such expert systems cannot generally use a fixed set of rules but rather need to learn to recognise patterns within complex sets of data. Techniques such as neural networks and fuzzy logic have been explored for this purpose (Chau, 2001). No doubt the number and quality of such systems will increase in the future. The following paragraphs describe how gait assessment is used for clinical decision making in a 'typical' laboratory. The details will, of course, differ from one laboratory to another, based on the skills and interests of the laboratory personnel, the facilities and equipment available, and the types of patient seen.

When the patient arrives at the facility informed consent is taken, a thorough history is then obtained and a physical examination is performed, by both a doctor, a physiotherapist, and sometimes others such as a prosthetist. Height, weight and a number of other measurements are made. The patient's gait is video-recorded, viewing the patient from both sides and from the front and back. The 'technological' element of the gait analysis is performed, using a television/computer kinematic system and one or more force platforms. The number of cameras used is dictated largely by economics. Ideally, at least six cameras should be used but three can give acceptable data, particularly if measurements are made from only one side of the body at a time. Most laboratories record surface EMG, either on muscles which are selected on a case-by-case basis or on a standard set, such as gluteus maximus, quadriceps (in particular rectus femoris), medial and lateral hamstrings, triceps surae, tibialis anterior and the hip adductors. Depending on the clinical condition, fine wire EMG of selected muscles may be recorded, either at the same time or later. For example, Gage et al. (1984) reported that where a hip flexion contracture is present, their laboratory routinely records fine wire EMG from the iliopsoas, however this is not common clinical practice. There is variation in the protocols used, with some facilities recording kinetic, kinematic and EMG data at the same time, whereas others find it more convenient to record EMG separately.

Since great variability may exist between one walk and another, any single walk may not be representative, particularly if the patient hesitates or momentarily loses their balance. For this reason, a number of walks are recorded and the results examined for consistency. Depending on the clinical status of the

Table 5.1 Common gait abnormalities, their possible causes and evidence required for confirmation

Foot slap at heel contact	Below normal dorsiflexor activity at heel contact	Below normal tibialis anterior EMG or dorsiflexor moment at heel contact
Forefoot or flatfoot initial contact	(a) Hyperactive plantarflexor activity in late swing (b) Structural limitation in ankle range (c) Short step length	(a) Above normal plantarflexor EMG in late swing (b) Decreased dorsiflexor range of motion (c) See (a–d) immediately below
Short step	(a) Weak push off prior to swing (b) Weak hip flexors at toe off and early swing (c) Excessive deceleration of leg in late swing (d) Above normal contralateral hip extensor activity during contralateral stance	(a) Below normal plantarflexor moment or power generation or EMG during push off (b) Below normal hip flexor moment or power or EMG during late push off and early swing (c) Above normal hamstring EMG or knee flexor moment or power absorption late in swing (d) Hyperactivity in EMG of contralateral hip extensors
Stiff-legged weightbearing	Above normal extensor activity at the ankle, knee or hip early in stance*	Above normal EMG activity or moments in hip extensors, knee extensors or plantarflexors early in stance
Stance phase with flexed but rigid knee	Above normal extensor activity in early and mid-stance at the ankle and hip, but with reduced knee extensor activity	Above normal EMG activity or moments in hip extensors and plantarflexors in early and mid-stance
Weak push off accompanied by observable pull off	Weak plantarflexor activity at push off. Normal, or above normal, hip flexor activity during late push off and early swing	Below normal plantarflexor EMG, moment or power during push off. Normal or above normal hip flexor EMG or moment or power during late push off and early swing
Hip hiking in swing (with or without circumduction of lower limb)	(a) Weak hip, knee or ankle dorsiflexor activity during swing (b) Overactive extensor synergy during swing	(a) Below normal tibialis anterior EMG or hip or knee flexors during swing (b) Above normal hip or knee extensor EMG or moment during swing
Trendelenburg gait	(a) Weak hip abductors (b) Overactive hip adductors	(a) Below normal EMG in hip abductors: gluteus medius and minimus, tensor fascia lata (b) Above normal EMG in hip adductors, adductor longus, magnus and brevis, and gracilis

*Note: there may be below normal extensor forces at one joint but only in the presence of abnormally high extensor forces at one or both of the other joints.
Reproduced with permission from Winter (1985).

patient, walks may be made under a number of different conditions, for example with and without shoes, with or without an orthosis, or using different walking aids. Activities such as rising from a chair or walking up and down steps can also be studied, however, it may not be possible to obtain force plate data.

Once preliminary reports on the history and physical examination have been prepared, the data processed and charts printed, the 'team' meets to discuss the case. The composition of the team varies considerably from one facility to another, but it would commonly consist of a doctor, a physiotherapist and a kinaesiologist or bio-engineer, with the optional addition of other doctors, physiotherapists, prosthetists, orthotists and podiatrists. Indeed, anyone with an interest in providing the best possible care for the patient may be invited to join the team to discuss a particular patient. In many facilities, the team includes the orthopaedic surgeon who will ultimately perform any necessary surgery.

The assessment begins with a careful review of the patient's history and the physical examinations by the doctor and physiotherapist. The gait video recording is watched frame by frame and discussed and notes are made for inclusion in a final report. The general gait parameters are noted to determine the degree of disability and the effects of any changes in conditions, such as orthoses or walking aids. Different gait analysis systems provide different amounts of technical data on the patient's gait and examination of the 'charts' can be a long and painstaking process. One of the most important parts of the assessment is to identify deviations from normal in the joint angles and to determine the cause of such deviations. This process is easier if joint moments and powers are available. Joint moments indicate in general terms which structures in the region of a joint are coming under tension and the degree of tension in them. Joint powers may help to discriminate between concentric muscle contraction, eccentric muscle contraction and passive tension in soft tissues. They can also distinguish between powerful and weak muscle contractions. The EMG also contributes to this process by identifying which muscles are electrically active and are thus candidates for developing tension at different times during the gait cycle.

Very briefly, interpretation of the gait analysis charts may involve the following steps. Commonly a comparison of the left to right sides is made when doing this.

1. *Joint angle:* what is the angle of a joint at a particular part of the gait cycle and in which direction is it moving?

2. *Joint moment:* what is the internal moment acting about the joint? This will indicate what muscles or ligaments are under tension and to what degree.

3. *Joint power:* what power generation or absorption is taking place? This would indicate concentric or eccentric contraction, or storage and release of energy by stretching elastic tissues.

4. *EMG:* what is the muscle electrical activity and is it consistent with the kinematic data?

At this time, a hypothesis is formed as to the detailed cause of any gait abnormalities present. This may indicate a need for further data, such as fine wire EMG recordings from other muscles (Fig. 5.1), and the patient may be asked to return for further tests. Having made a detailed diagnosis of the patient's functional problems, the team decides on an appropriate form of treatment. This could involve treatment through physiotherapy, orthotics, surgery,

drug treatment, or a combination of these. In such cases, the final stage of assessment would be an 'examination under anaesthesia' when appropriate, made just prior to the commencement of surgery. The muscle relaxant used with the anaesthetic abolishes spasticity and makes it possible to distinguish between structural abnormalities, such as contractures, and the effects of muscle tension. If the treatment selected involves drug treatment, physiotherapy or the use of an orthosis, the patient would be monitored during the course of such treatment, to determine whether the initial decisions were appropriate.

Once treatment has been carried out and after a suitable recovery period, a further gait assessment is often performed. The purpose of this is firstly to determine the success of the treatment and secondly to decide whether the patient would benefit from further surgery, physiotherapy or the prescription of an orthosis. It also gives the clinical team the opportunity to perform a critical review of the original diagnosis and treatment plan, to decide whether the correct decisions were made. If an error has been made, it is important to recognise it and to learn from it, to prevent it from happening again. There is usually no change in EMG postoperatively and the main criteria for determining the success (or otherwise) of treatment are the general gait parameters and the joint rotations. In subjects in whom it can be measured from the kinematic data, the estimated external work of walking (EEWW) may also be used as a measure of improvement. According to Gage, total body energy consumption is the best measure of the success of treatment whereas Perry (2010) uses three criteria to gauge success: walking speed, energy consumption and cosmesis.

Diagnosis of abnormal gait

Most patients undergoing gait assessment have already been diagnosed, as far as the principal disease or condition affecting them is concerned. In such cases, gait assessment is carried out to make a more detailed diagnosis, relating to the exact state of particular joints and muscles. On occasion, however, a patient is seen in whom the cause of an abnormal gait is not clear.

A number of apparently abnormal gait patterns are, in fact, habits rather than the result of underlying pathology and the techniques of gait analysis may be useful to identify them. Since any pathology affecting the locomotor system generally reduces a person's

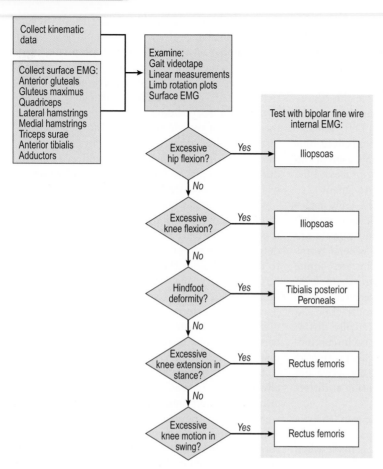

Fig. 5.1 • Gait assessment flowchart, used for selecting muscles for testing with fine wire EMG (©1988 IEEE. Reprinted, with permission, from Davis RB, Clinical gait analysis. IEEE Engineering in Medicine and Biology Magazine September: 35–40).

ability to alter their gait pattern, a variable gait may be suggestive of a habit pattern and a highly reproducible gait may suggest a pathological process. However, the assessment must take many other factors into account, including the possibility of a pathological process which includes an element of variability, such as ataxia or athetosis. One unusual application of gait analysis is to distinguish between a gait abnormality due to a genuine neuromuscular cause and one due to a psychogenic cause, such as may be seen in cases of malingering (Wesdock et al., 2003).

An example of the use of gait assessment to differentiate between pathological gaits and habit patterns is in the diagnosis of toe walking. Some children prefer to walk on their toes, rather than on the whole foot, in a pattern known as 'idiopathic toe walking'. It is important, but also quite difficult, to be able to differentiate between this relatively harmless and self-limiting condition and more serious conditions, such as cerebral palsy. Hicks et al. (1988) stated that earlier attempts to establish the diagnosis, using EMG alone, had not been successful. In their study, they compared the gait kinematics of seven idiopathic toe walkers and seven children with mild spastic diplegia. There was a clear difference between the two groups in the pattern of sagittal plane knee and ankle motion. Both groups had initial contact either by the flat foot or by toe strike but in the case of the toe walkers, this was due to ankle plantarflexion, whereas in the children with cerebral palsy it was due to knee flexion. There were also other differences between the two groups, suggesting that gait assessment would be very helpful in making a differential diagnosis.

Documentation of a patient's condition

Although clinical decision making is the most direct way in which gait assessment may be used to help an individual patient, there are also instances when simply documenting the current state of a patient's gait may be of value. For some purposes, such documentation may be needed only on a single occasion, where the aim is to quantify a patient's disability. For other purposes, a series of gait assessments over a period of time may be used to monitor either progress or deterioration.

As part of the overall assessment of a patient with a disability, a clinician may require more detail about how well they walk. This type of gait assessment may be directly intended for use in clinical decision making, but it is sometimes performed speculatively, in case it should reveal a treatable cause for the patient's walking disorder.

Gait assessment is frequently used to document the progress of a patient undergoing some form of treatment. The results of the assessment may be used to identify areas where the treatment is ineffective or it may define an end point for stopping treatment, when progress appears to have ceased. Another use of this type of serial assessment is to convince the patient or their relatives that progress has been made, when they think it has not. An objective form of monitoring progress is particularly important for use in the evaluation of novel and controversial methods of treatment, where the enthusiasm of the investigators has been known to lead to errors of judgement!

Gait assessment may form part of the overall documentation of a number of medical conditions that involve the locomotor system. A deterioration in gait with the passage of time may be detected early, allowing remedial action to be taken. It may also identify clinical signs which should be looked for in other cases of the same condition, particularly if it is very uncommon.

Conditions benefiting from gait assessment

A large number of diseases affect the neuromuscular and musculoskeletal systems and may thus lead to disorders of gait. Among the most important are:

1. Cerebral palsy
2. Parkinsonism
3. Muscular dystrophy
4. Osteoarthritis
5. Rheumatoid arthritis
6. Lower limb amputation
7. Stroke
8. Head injury

9. Spinal cord injury
10. Myelodysplasia
11. Multiple sclerosis.

While it is possible that gait assessment may benefit a person affected by any one of these conditions, it is clear that greater benefits are possible in some pathologies than in others. The next two chapters will consider neurological and musculoskeletal conditions for which there is good evidence that gait assessment is worthwhile.

Future developments

Advanced techniques to quantify deviation from normality

There has been a recent surge of interest in trying to meet the requirements of clinicians and clients/patients looking for simple measures of gait which encapsulate the rich information content of a gait analysis, as opposed to detailed and lengthy gait reports typically generated by gait laboratories. The two opposing sides of simplicity and complexity represent the two approaches to abnormal human gait. On one side the clinician's and patient's result-oriented approach is that they aim to make gait more normal and so their focus is on the overall quality of gait (Kelly et al., 1997). On the other side the gait analyst's approach is to search for the causes underlying gait deviations by analysing gait quantitatively. Interventions prescribed by clinicians are based on the findings of the quantitative approach but are ultimately aimed at improving the quality of gait and so there is an incompatibility between the questions oriented to gait quality, and the answers derived from quantitative data. This incompatibility, however, can be resolved considering that the quantitative representation of a gait abnormality inherently contains a measure of deviation from normality distributed across a large number of gait curves. Therefore we need an appropriate method to extract a measure of gait quality from the quantitative gait data.

Only a few methods have been described which may bridge the gap between the quantitative and qualitative approach to gait by calculating overall quality measures derived from quantitative data. The normalcy index (NI) (Schutte et al., 2000) is a single number representing the deviation between a subject's gait and an average normal profile, calculated from 16 discrete gait variables measured by routine clinical gait analysis (timing of foot off, walking speed, cadence, walking distance, mean and peak angles of the pelvis, hip, knee and ankle joints in selected planes). The Gillette gait index (GGI) (Romei et al., 2004, 2005; Theologis et al., 2005) based on Schutte and co-workers' NI was shown to be a reliable method sensitive enough to separate different pathological gait patterns. The GGI has been extensively evaluated (Romei et al., 2004; Wren et al., 2007) and has been used in gait analysis research to test if an intervention leads to improved gait function (e.g. Gorton et al., 2009). A similar index described by Tingley et al. (2002) considers multiple joint angle curves simultaneously and produces a single score that enables the classification of children as normal, unusual or abnormal.

Gait indices quantify the deviation of gait from normal and so can be regarded as measures of gait quality. Their use, however, does not extend to identifying the causes of gait problems because the single score characterises the patient's gait as a whole and therefore it cannot be related to when the deviations occur in the gait cycle or to which of the joints were the source of the deviation. A recognised limitation of the GGI is that the choice of the 16 kinematic parameters used to calculate the index was based on the subjective judgement of clinicians and so may not be the best possible set of parameters for different pathologies. Indeed, several authors (Romei et al., 2004, 2005; Schutte et al., 2000; Theologis et al., 2005) suggested the inclusion of additional gait variables to the GGI to further improve its potential.

The above limitations of gait indices, that they contribute little to establishing the cause–effect links underlying gait problems and that they are based only on a subset of the gait data, have been addressed in the work of Barton et al. (2003, 2007), Schwartz and Rozumalski (2008) and Baker et al. (2009). Barton et al. (2003) described the use of a 'self-organising neural network' to quantify the quality of gait. This allows a set of kinematic and kinetic variables taken from normal gait to 'train' the network, resulting in an autonomous definition of normality. The neural network can then be used to describe how far a patient's gait is from normality. An advantage of this technique is that it allows deviations from normality to be calculated at all points in the gait cycle, and it determines which joints contribute most to the deviations. Schwartz and Rozumalski (2008) addressed the limitations of the GGI by developing a new and comprehensive measure of gait pathology.

A set of 15 gait features were extracted from nine joint angle curves of a large number of patients and typically developing control children to define the full spectrum of normal and pathological gait. The distance of a patient from the mean of controls in the 15 dimensional gait feature space was termed the gait deviation index (GDI). Validation of the GDI showed good agreement with measures of movement function and sub-types of pathologies. Baker et al. (2009), inspired by the GDI, developed the gait profile score (GPS) which is the root mean square difference between a patient's data and the mean of controls, taken over several kinematic variables along the entire gait cycle. Through validation against the GGI, GDI, and measures of motor function in a large number of patients, the GPS was found to be a closely related alternative to the GDI.

Barton et al. (2010) used artificial neural networks as an alternative to conventional analysis of large number of joint and moment patterns. Even without any knowledge of the pathological conditions in the population, the self-organising map (SOM) artificial neural network (Kohonen, 1988, 2001) was able to quantify the deviation from normality by calculating the distance between abnormal and normal patterns. Joint angles, recorded from typically developing children over one gait cycle, were used to train a SOM which then generated movement deviation profile (MDP) curves showing the deviation of patients' gait from normality. The mean MDP over the gait cycle showed a high correlation ($r^2 = 0.927$) with the GDI, a statistically significant difference between groups of patients with a range of functional levels (Gillette functional assessment questionnaire walking scale 7–10) and a trend of increasing values for patients with cerebral palsy through hemiplegia I–IV, diplegia, triplegia and quadriplegia. Therefore the MDP can be regarded as an alternative method of processing complex biomechanical data, potentially supporting clinical interpretation. A stand-alone program which can be used to calculate the MDP from gait data is available as an electronic addendum accompanying the paper by Barton et al. (2010) in *Human Movement Science* and also from http://www.staff.ljmu.ac.uk/spsgbart/MDP.htm (Fig. 5.2).

Comprehending a full gait report may be too challenging but a single number gait index may hide details needed to find the cause of gait problems. A variety of related but different methods with firm theoretical justifications are now available, aiding the interpretation of gait data. Free software tools are accessible to calculate the GDI and GPS using Microsoft Excel,

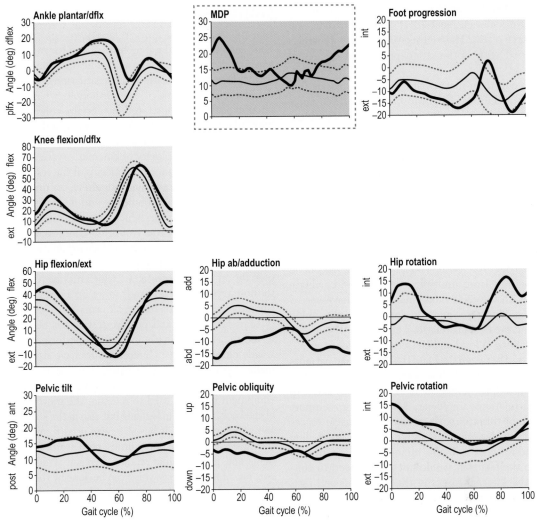

Fig. 5.2 • The movement deviation profile (MDP) inserted in the conventional presentation of gait kinematics. Note that the axes and the presentation of a patient's MDP curve over the mean and SD of controls is identical to the other curves. The MDP chart (surrounded by a dotted line) summarises the other nine angle curves (bold curves) and shows the timing and extent of deviations from normality (thin curves) during the gait cycle (Barton et al., 2010).

and the MDP with a stand-alone Windows program. Future research is now needed to identify the benefits and disadvantages of simplification through further validation against clinical criteria.

Modelling muscle forces and EMG-assisted models

Gait analysis has advanced significantly since joint moments and powers became routinely available. What would be of even more value, if it could be provided, would be knowledge of the forces in the different structures in and around the joints. The use of mathematical modelling permits estimates to be made of forces in tendons and ligaments and across articular surfaces. Unfortunately, a large number of unknown factors are involved, particularly the internal moments generated by different muscles and the extent of any co-contraction by antagonistic muscles. For this reason, such calculations can only be approximate but they may nonetheless be extremely valuable, particularly in clinical and biomechanical research. One example is Motek's Human Body

Model, which calculates multiple muscle forces from three-dimensional (3D) kinematic data and dual force plates. The method uses inverse dynamics combined with optimisation performed by neural networks.

The output of mathematical models may be further refined using EMG. Most models offer a range of possible solutions, based on different combinations of active muscles. Even though it is not generally possible to convert EMG signals directly into muscle contraction force, the knowledge that a muscle is either inactive, contracting a little or contracting strongly may make it possible to eliminate at least some of the possible model solutions and thereby to improve the reliability of the results. These models try to account for changes in musculotendon length, velocity, and the amount of electrical activity for both concentric and eccentric contractions from multiple muscles, and correlate these with the joint moments. Results have varied considerably from joint to joint with the ankle showing the best correlations of up to 0.91 for normal walking (Lloyd and Besier, 2003; Bogey et al., 2005) and between 0.87 and 0.92 for stroke patients (Shao et al., 2009), however, as we consider the more proximal joints such as the knee and hip the correlations are lower. Most authors support the use of this approach to estimate muscle forces during gait, however research using such modelling techniques is still in the minority. This is mainly due to the fact that we do not always need to consider the internal forces in the tendinous and ligamentous structures as these are rarely the primary outcome measures in gait assessment.

Conclusion

Gait analysis has had a long history and for much of this time it has remained an academic discipline with little practical application. This situation has now changed and the value of the methodology has been unequivocally demonstrated in certain conditions, particularly cerebral palsy. We are seeing a decrease in the cost and improvements in the ease of use of an ever-increasing complexity of kinematic systems and an increasing acceptance by clinicians of the results of gait analysis. This trend will hopefully continue, so that the use of these techniques will increase, both in those conditions for which its value is already recognised and in a variety of other conditions.

Although the current text has focused on gait analysis, this type of measurement equipment may also be used for other purposes – a fact which may be relevant to those trying to obtain funds to set up a gait analysis laboratory! The use of force platforms and kinematic systems for balance and posture testing has been referred to, as has their use in studying performance in a wide range of sports. Clinical studies have also been made of people standing up, sitting down, starting and stopping walking, ascending and descending stairs. The equipment has been used to measure the movements of the back, not only in walking but also in the standing and sitting positions. It has also been used to monitor the movements of the upper limbs, both in athetoid patients and in ergonomic studies of reach. Walking is only one of many things which can be done by the musculoskeletal system. It is only sensible to broaden our horizons and to use the power of the modern measurement systems to study a wide range of other activities.

References

Baker, R., McGinley, J.L., Schwartz, M.H., et al., 2009. The gait profile score and movement analysis profile. Gait Posture 30, 265–269.

Barton, G.J., Lees, A., Lisboa, P., et al., 2003. Visualisation of gait quality using self organising artificial neural networks. Gait Posture 18 (Suppl. 2), 119.

Barton, G., Lisboa, P., Lees, A., et al., 2007. Gait quality assessment using self-organising artificial neural networks. Gait Posture 25, 374–379.

Barton, G.J., Hawken, M.B., Scott, M., et al., (2010) Movement deviation profile: a measure of distance from normality using a self organising neural network. Invited paper in Special Issue on Network Approaches in Complex Environments, Hum. Mov. Sci. http://dx.doi.org/10.1016/j.humov.2010.06.003 (accessed 30.08.11.).

Bogey, R.A., Perry, J., Gitter, A.J., 2005. An EMG-to-force processing approach for determining ankle muscle forces during normal human gait. IEEE Transactions on Neural Systems and Rehabilitation Engineering 13 (3), 302–310.

Chau, T., 2001. A review of analytical techniques for gait data. Part 1: fuzzy, statistical and fractal methods. Gait Posture 13, 49–66.

Davis, R.B., 1988. Clinical gait analysis. IEEE Eng. Med. Biol. Mag. September, 35–40.

Gage, J.R., 1983. Gait analysis for decision-making in cerebral palsy. Bull. Hosp. Jt. Dis. Orthop. Inst. 43, 147–163.

Gage, J.R., Fabian, D., Hicks, R., et al., 1984. Pre- and postoperative gait analysis in patients with spastic diplegia: a preliminary report. J. Pediatr. Orthop. 4, 715–725.

Gorton 3rd., G.E., Abel, M.F., Oeffinger, D.J., et al., 2009. A prospective cohort study of the effects of lower extremity orthopaedic surgery on outcome measures in ambulatory children with cerebral palsy. J. Pediatr. Orthop. 29, 903–909.

Hicks, R., Durinick, N., Gage, J.R., 1988. Differentiation of idiopathic toe-walking and cerebral palsy. J. Pediatr. Orthop. 8, 160–163.

Kelly, I.P., O'Regan, M., Jenkinson, A., O'Brien, T., 1997. The quality assessment of walking in cerebral palsy. Gait and Posture, 5, 70–74.

Kohonen, T., 1988. Self-organisation and Associative Memory. Springer, Berlin.

Kohonen, T., 2001. Self-organizing Maps. Springer, Berlin.

Lloyd, D.G., Besier, T.F., 2003. An EMG-driven musculoskeletal model to estimate muscle forces and knee joint moments in vivo. J. Biomech. 36, 765–776.

Perry, J., 2010. Gait analysis: Normal and pathological function. Slack Incorporated, Thorofare, NJ.

Romei, M., Galli, M., Motta, F., et al., 2004. Use of the normalcy index for the evaluation of gait pathology. Gait Posture 19, 85–90.

Romei, M., Galli, M., Motta, F., et al., 2005. Reply to 'Letter to the Editor'. Gait Posture 22, 378.

Rose, G.K., 1983. Clinical gait assessment: a personal view. J. Med. Eng. Technol. 7, 273–279.

Schutte, L.M., Narayanan, U., Stout, J.L., et al., 2000. An index for quantifying deviations from normal gait. Gait Posture 11, 25–31.

Schwartz, M.H., Rozumalski, A., 2008. The gait deviation index: a new comprehensive index of gait pathology. Gait Posture 28, 351–357.

Shao, Q., Bassett, D.N., Manal, K., et al., 2009. An EMG-driven model to estimate muscle forces and joint moments in stroke patients. Comput. Biol. Med. 39 (12), 1083–1088.

Theologis, T., Thompson, N., Harrington, M., 2005. Letter to the editor. Gait Posture 22, 377.

Tingley, M., Wilson, C., Biden, E., et al., 2002. An index to quantify normality of gait in young children. Gait Posture 16, 149–158.

Wesdock, K., Blair, S., Masiello, G., et al., 2003. Psychogenic gait: when it is and when it isn't – correlating the physical exam with dynamic gait data. In: Gait and Clinical Movement Analysis Society, Eighth Annual Meeting, Wilmington, Delaware, USA, pp. 279–280.

Winter, D.A., 1985. Concerning the scientific basis for the diagnosis of pathological gait and for rehabilitation protocols. Physiother. Can. 37, 245–252.

Wren, T.A., Do, K.P., Hara, R., et al., 2007. Gillette Gait Index as a gait analysis summary measure: comparison with qualitative visual assessments of overall gait. J. Pediatr. Orthop. 27, 765–768.

Further reading

Berchuck, M., Andriacchi, T.P., Bach, B.R., et al., 1990. Gait adaptations by patients who have a deficient anterior cruciate ligament. J. Bone Joint Surg. Am. 72, 871–877.

Cavanagh, P.R., Hennig, E.M., Rodgers, M.M., et al., 1985. The measurement of pressure distribution on the plantar surface of diabetic feet. In: Whittle, M., Harris, D. (Eds.), Biomechanical Measurement in Orthopaedic Practice. Clarendon Press, Oxford, pp. 159–166.

Davis, R.B., 1988. Clinical gait analysis. IEEE Eng. Med. Biol. Mag. September, 35–40.

Harrington, E.D., Lin, R.S., Gage, J.R., 1984. Use of the anterior floor reaction orthosis in patients with cerebral palsy. Orthotics and Prosthetics 37, 34–42.

Hicks, R., Tashman, S., Cary, J.M., et al., 1985. Swing phase control with knee friction in juvenile amputees. J. Orthop. Res. 3, 198–201.

Jefferson, R.J., Whittle, M.W., 1989. Biomechanical assessment of unicompartmental knee arthroplasty, total condylar arthroplasty and tibial osteotomy. Clin. Biomech. (Bristol, Avon) 4, 232–242.

Kohonen, T., 1988. Self-organisation and Associative Memory. Springer, Berlin.

Kohonen, T., 2001. Self-organizing Maps. Springer, Berlin.

Lehmann, J.F., Condon, S.M., Price, R., et al., 1987. Gait abnormalities in hemiplegia: their correction by ankle-foot orthoses. Arch. Phys. Med. Rehabil. 68, 763–771.

Lord, M., Reynolds, D.P., Hughes, J.R., 1986. Foot pressure measurement: a review of clinical findings. J. Biomed. Eng. 8, 283–294.

Molloy, M., McDowell, B.C., Kerr, C., et al., 2010. Further evidence of validity of the Gait Deviation Index. Gait Posture 31, 479–482.

New York University, 1986. Lower Limb Orthotics. New York University Postgraduate Medical School, New York, NY.

Õunpuu, S., Davis, R.B., DeLuca, P.A., 1996. Joint kinetics: methods, interpretation and treatment decision-making in children with cerebral palsy and myelomeningocele. Gait Posture 4, 62–78.

Prodromos, C.C., Andriacchi, T.P., Galante, J.O., 1985. A relationship between gait and clinical changes following high tibial osteotomy. J. Bone Joint Surg. Am. 67, 1188–1194.

Roberts, C.S., Rash, G.S., Honaker, J.T., et al., 1999. A deficient anterior cruciate ligament does not lead to quadriceps avoidance gait. Gait Posture 10, 189–199.

Tashman, S., Hicks, R., Jendrzejczyk, D.J., 1985. Evaluation of a prosthetic shank with variable inertial properties. Clinical Prosthetics and Orthotics 9, 23–28.

Waters, R.L., Garland, D.E., Perry, J., et al., 1979. Stiff-legged gait in hemiplegia: surgical correction. J. Bone Joint Surg. Am. 61, 927–933.

Gait assessment of neurological disorders

6

Richard Baker   Nancy Fell   Jim Richards   Cathie Smith

The aim of this chapter is to provide examples of how gait analysis can be used to determine the severity, progression and the efficacy of non-surgical, surgical and pharmaceutical management of neurological disorders. This chapter will consider several common disorders and their management, including cerebral palsy, hemiplegia, Parkinson's disease and muscular dystrophy.

Gait assessment in cerebral palsy

Definition, causes and prevalence

Cerebral palsy is now defined as a group of permanent disorders of the development of movement and posture which can be attributed to brain damage to the fetus or infant (Rosenbaum et al., 2007). The condition is different from other forms of brain damage such as stroke or traumatic brain injury because it happens while the brain is still developing and this affects the subsequent neurological and musculoskeletal development of the child. The motor disorders of cerebral palsy are often accompanied by disturbances of sensation, perception, cognition, communication and behaviour, and by epilepsy. Cerebral palsy is the commonest cause of physical disability affecting children in the developed world with a prevalence of around 2 cases for every 1000 live births (Stanley et al., 2000). Figures for other parts of the world are difficult to ascertain but it is generally assumed to be at least as prevalent.

The brain damage is much more common in infants born prematurely but the precise cause is unknown in the majority of cases. The ultimate cause is a failure of the oxygen supply to an area of the developing brain which may be a consequence of damage to the blood vessels, such as haemorrhage or embolism, or a more general drop in fetal blood pressure. The brain damage, once it has occurred, is static and will not get any better or any worse. The clinical manifestations, however, will continue to develop and change as the child grows and matures. This is particularly true of the musculoskeletal manifestations of cerebral palsy, which are very important in determining whether and how people with the condition will walk.

Classification

Gross motor function classification system

The principal means of classifying children with cerebral palsy is with the Gross Motor Function Classification System GMFCS (Palisano et al., 1997 and 2000). This is, essentially a five-point scale reflecting the severity of the condition as it affects motor function. There are different definitions for different age groups but that for 6–12 year olds is the most relevant to gait analysts (Table 6.1). It can be seen that most children who are suitable for gait analysis will be of levels I–III. More recently descriptors for 12–18 year olds have been produced (Palisano et al., 2008). These are similar to those in Table 6.1 but

Table 6.1 Gross Motor Function Classification System for children aged 6–12 years

Level I	Children walk indoors and outdoors and climb stairs without limitation. Children perform gross motor skills including running and jumping, but speed, balance and coordination are impaired
Level II	Children walk indoors and outdoors and climb stairs holding onto a railing but experience limitations walking on uneven surfaces and inclines and walking in crowds or confined spaces and with long distances
Level III	Children walk indoors and outdoors on a level surface with an assistive mobility device and may climb stairs holding onto a railing. Children may use a wheelchair for mobility when travelling for long distances or outdoors over uneven terrain.
Level IV	Children use methods of mobility that usually require adult assistance. They may continue to walk for short distances with physical assistance at home but rely on wheeled mobility (pushed by adult or operate a powered chair) outdoors, at school and in the community
Level V	Physical impairment restricts voluntary control of movement and the ability to maintain anti-gravity head and trunk posture. All areas of motor function are limited. Children have no means of independent mobility and are transported by adults

allow for some deterioration in motor ability that occurs in late childhood. While gait analysis is most often used for children with cerebral palsy it is worth remembering that cerebral palsy is a life-long condition, with between 25% and 50% of adults reporting further deterioration in walking ability in early adulthood (Day et al., 2007; Jahnsen et al., 2004; Murphy et al., 1995).

Classification by motor disorder and topography

The brain damage that causes cerebral palsy can affect the nervous system in several different ways. In about 85% of people the major limitation is spasticity, which leads to over activity in specific muscles. A further 7% are dyskinetic (dystonic-athetoid) having mixed muscle tone (high or low), which leads to slow sinuous movements superimposed on the intended motor pattern. Another 5% have ataxia which leads to rapid jerky movements and affects balance and depth perception. People with dyskinesia or ataxia tend to have very variable gait patterns, which can limit the usefulness of clinical gait analysis. Outcomes of orthopaedic surgery in people with dyskinesia can be unpredictable. Most children attending for clinical gait analysis are therefore those with a predominantly spastic motor type.

Before the advent of the GMFCS, the primary classification of children with cerebral palsy was with respect to the areas of the body that were most affected. *Hemiplegia* refers to one side of the body being affected including an arm and leg on the same side. *Diplegia* refers to the involvement of both legs and *quadriplegia* to involvement of all four limbs. *Monoplegia* (involvement of one limb) and *triplegia* (involvement of three limbs) are also used. Many children do not fall neatly into these categories and the distinction between quadriplegia and diplegia is rarely clear-cut; many diplegic individuals are affected much more on one side than the other. Such issues have led to recent advice that such terms be discontinued until they are defined more precisely. *Unilateral* and *bilateral motor involvements* are now the preferred terms for children who can walk with *total body involvement* being used for non-walkers. Having said this, the original terms are still in widespread use.

Classification by gait pattern

There have been several attempts to classify cerebral palsy on the basis of the gait pattern (Dobson et al., 2007). Some confusion has arisen because several authors have chosen to re-define terms used by previous authors and it is not always clear which classification system is being referred to by which term. Two classifications for spastic hemiplegic gait have been proposed (Hullin et al., 1996; Winters et al., 1987) of which Winters et al. is more commonly used. This is described in Figure 6.1 and Table 6.2. There is some confusion in how this is applied clinically. The original paper refers exclusively to the sagittal plane and is based purely on the gait pattern. It is not at all uncommon to hear clinicians incorporating consideration of the transverse plane

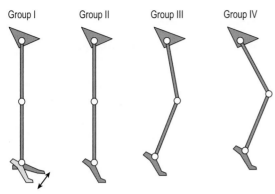

Fig. 6.1 • Common gait patterns in hemiplegic cerebral palsy (reproduced with permission and copyright © of the British Editorial Society of Bone and Joint Surgery. (Rodda et al., 2004).

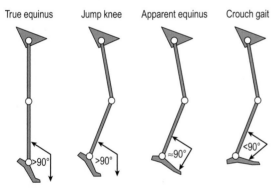

Fig. 6.2 • Common gait patterns in spastic diplegic cerebral palsy (Rodda et al., 2004).

(particularly at the hip) and inferences about the nature of the underlying pathology (rather than just the gait pattern) in classifying children. Agreement between clinicians in applying this classification is substantial (Dobson et al., 2006). A more recent population-based study suggested that groups I, II and IV are far more common than group III.

Classifications of gait patterns in spastic diplegia are less clear cut. One example is the classification by Rodda et al. (2004) in which the whole gait pattern is described (Fig. 6.2 and Table 6.3). There is particular confusion with regard to a number of terms that different people have chosen to define differently. Sutherland and Davids (1993), for example defined 'jump' as referring to a pattern in which the knee is flexed in early stance but extends rapidly in a pattern reminiscent of jumping. Rodda et al. (2004) used the same term to refer to a posture of flexed knee and plantarflexed ankle in late stance. 'Crouch' gait is another term that has been defined differently by a range of authors. Many studies simply use the term to refer to a gait pattern exhibiting knee flexion of no less than a certain value (30° is commonly used) throughout stance. Gage et al. (2009) used a kinetic definition for patterns in which the internal knee moment is extensor throughout stance, whereas Rodda et al. (2004) required ankle dorsiflexon as well as knee flexion.

Classification by gait pattern does not give the whole picture. The two most commonly used schemes are based on sagittal plane data only (Rodda et al., 2004; Winters et al., 1987). Winters et al. proposed their classification system for people who had had no previous orthopaedic intervention

Table 6.2 Classification of gait patterns in hemiplegia*

Group I	Ankle equinus in the swing phase of gait due to underactivity of the ankle dorsiflexors in relation to the plantarflexors
Group II	Plantarflexion throughout stance and swing from either static or dynamic contracture of the triceps surae. Knee is often forced into slight hyperextension in middle or late stance
Group III	Findings of type II with reduced range of knee flexion/extension. Reference is now common to sub-types IIIa: reduced knee extension during stance, and IIIb: hyperextension in stance and reduced flexion in swing
Group IV	Findings of type III with involvement of the hip musculature†

*Summary by Thompson et al. (2002) of original by Winters et al. (1987).
†In the original paper, in which measurements were restricted to the sagittal plane, this was attributed to flexor and adductor involvement. A three-dimensional analysis would almost certainly have included increased internal rotation

Table 6.3 Common gait patterns in spastic diplegic cerebral palsy (Rodda et al., 2004)

Group I	The ankle is in equinus. The knee extends fully or goes into mild recurvatum. The hip extends fully and the pelvis is within the normal range or tilted anteriorly
Group II	The ankle is in equinus, particularly in late stance. The knee and hip are excessively flexed in early stance and then extend to a variable degree in late stance, but never reach full extension. The pelvis is either within the normal range or tilted anteriorly
Group III	The ankle has a normal range but the knee and hip are excessively flexed throughout stance. The pelvis is normal or tilted anteriorly
Group IV	The ankle is excessively dorsiflexed throughout stance and the knee and hip are excessively flexed. The pelvis is in the normal range or tilted posteriorly

and it is not clear how much value the scheme has for people who have had surgery. Rodda et al. did not discuss how surgery, or other interventions, would affect classification by gait pattern. There is considerable variability within grades and some people clearly have patterns on the boundary between one grade and the next. Indeed two studies which include data that can be used to infer whether natural groupings exist (Dobson, 2007; Rozumalski and Schwartz, 2009) would suggest, on the contrary, that gait patterns vary continuously across a multi-dimensional spectrum and groupings will only ever be a rather gross guide to the general pattern of movement. They can, however, still be useful in giving an overall impression of the person's gait pattern particularly if full instrumented gait analysis is not available. A full gait analysis is still essential if we want to be specific about how a person is walking and what is causing them to do so in a particular manner.

Impairments

An *impairment* is something that is wrong with a person's body structures or the way they function (World Health Organization (WHO), 2001). Examples of impairments include the loss of a limb or loss of vision. These can be complex in people with cerebral palsy. Primary impairments are direct consequences of the brain damage, and thus affect basic neurological function, whereas secondary impairments are indirect consequences arising from the effects of altered neurology on other structures over a long period of time. Thus muscles may become contracted or bones misaligned. Impairments generally fall into four broad categories: spasticity, weakness, muscle contracture and bony malalignment.

Spasticity

The term 'spasticity' means different things to different people. Most clinicians working with people with cerebral palsy[1] tend to use it to refer to a very specific 'velocity-dependent increase in tonic stretch reflexes, with exaggerated tendon jerks resulting from hyperexcitability of the stretch reflex' (Lance, 1980). In other words if a tendon is stretched rapidly then its muscle will become active. Depending on the severity of the spasticity this might be for a short period and the muscle may thus show phasic, but inappropriate activity throughout the gait cycle, or for a longer period in which case the muscle may be inappropriately active throughout the gait cycle. This stretch reflex is present in all of us but in most people is suppressed by signals originating in the brain and passing down the spinal column (descending control). In people with cerebral palsy the brain damage reduces the capacity to send such signals and the reflexes are effectively out of control. Thus, although it is common to hear reference to 'spastic muscles', spasticity is really a property of the nervous system.

In cerebral palsy spasticity commonly affects some muscles more than others. In particular the bi- and multiarticular muscles appear to be susceptible (Gage et al., 2009). Thus spasticity is commonly found in the gastrocnemius, hamstrings, rectus femoris and psoas muscles. In more severely affected children, spasticity of the monoarticular hip adductors is a particular issue.

---

[1] It is worth noting that many other clinicians use 'spasticity' in a much broader sense to cover a wider range of neurological signs.

Spasticity, so tightly defined, is not the only alteration to neurological function. In some people with cerebral palsy, particularly those most severely affected, there can be inappropriate muscle activity in the absence of movement as well, and this is generally referred to as *resting tone*. Dystonia and ataxia are also essentially the manifestation of neurological impairments.

Muscle contracture

Spasticity occurs in a wide range of conditions and in most of these the muscles affected are susceptible to develop *contractures*. In these the passive length of the muscle and its tendon are reduced and this leads to a restriction in the range of movement that is available at the joints. Most children with cerebral palsy are relatively free from contractures at birth and in infancy and then develop them through childhood. They are commonly named by the position they are held in: for example, a flexion contracture of the knee means that the knee is held in some degree of flexion and cannot fully extend, with the most commonly seen contractures including knee flexion, ankle plantarflexion and hip flexion.

The mechanisms by which contractures develop are not fully understood. In relation to children with cerebral palsy it is quite common to hear contractures talked about as a failure of normal growth, where the bone keeps on growing but the muscle does not. This cannot be the full picture, as some children, particularly those with hemiplegia, can develop contractures over a short period of time which are too severe to be explained simply by failure of growth. Contractures are also common in many adults who have spasticity (in conditions such as stroke). Another common belief is that contractures are a result of immobilisation, which is supported by some early clinical and animal work suggesting that this reduces the length of the muscle fibres (Shortland et al., 2002). Again though, there are many other conditions in which immobilisation of muscles is much more complete than in cerebral palsy, but such severe contractures do not develop. More recent work suggests that a reduction in muscle belly length through shortening of the aponeuroses is much more significant than any reduction in fibre length (Shortland et al., 2002), but no mechanism has been proposed for this. In summary, the development of contractures is probably related to failure of growth, immobilisation and the consequences of spasticity but the relative contributions of these factors remain unknown.

Weakness

It is only relatively recently that the effect of muscle weakness on the gait of people with cerebral palsy has been fully acknowledged. Wiley and Damiano (1998) surveyed the strength of children with cerebral palsy and demonstrated that muscle weakness is also important with the gluteal muscles with the plantarflexors also being particularly weak with respect to those of age-matched able-bodied children. Muscle weakness can arise either because of the anatomy and physiology of the muscles or through reduced neural activity to stimulate contraction. Despite cerebral palsy being an essentially neurological problem there have been few investigations to establish the relative proportions of the muscular and neurological components of weakness.

The weakness has generally been attributed to a muscle's reduced physiological cross-sectional area attributed to short muscle belly length and may therefore be strongly related to the development of contracture in both spastic hemiplegia and diplegia (Elder et al., 2003; Fry et al., 2007). The clinical picture does not always agree with this, with some muscles appearing to be quite weak without evidence of contracture. It is also known, however, that there is more extra-cellular material of lower quality than in normal muscle. Recent evidence suggests that these changes are quite different from those that arise simply through either chronic stimulation or disuse (Foran et al., 2005) but, as with the development of contracture, the underlying mechanisms are not understood. During movement there is a further factor in that contractures or specific walking patterns may result in muscle fibres functioning away from their optimal length to generate contractile force. The clinical picture appears to be that the muscles get weaker with age with respect to those of children without cerebral palsy. A particular issue arises in late childhood and early adolescent when weight increases rapidly and relative weakness becomes significant.

Bony malalignment (and capsular contracture)

Children with cerebral palsy are also susceptible to developing malalignment of the bones. Anteversion of the femur is the most common example of this. It is essentially a twist somewhere along the shaft of the femur which results in the femoral neck pointing too far forwards in relation to the knee joint axis. Although it is commonly referred to as a developmental deformity it is actually a result of persistence of the original bony alignment. At birth most children have anteversion of about 40° but this reduces in normal growth to about 10° at skeletal maturity. This reduction does not occur in many children with cerebral palsy. It is not uncommon for the tibia to be twisted externally along its shaft, *tibial torsion*, and malalignment of the bones of the foot, particularly the calcaneus is also common. In more severely affected children spinal, thoracic and upper limb deformities are also common.

As with the other impairments the precise mechanisms are unclear but at least three factors need to be considered. Bones grow in length at the *growth plates*. Most long bones have a growth plate proximally and distally. The rate at which the bones grow is determined by the stress exerted across the growth plate. In areas of the growth plate across which large compressive stresses are exerted, longitudinal growth will be suppressed and elsewhere growth may be stimulated. Thus normal bone growth requires normal stress distributions. Walking is believed to be a major contributor to such stresses and thus if children do not walk normally the bones will not grow normally. *Remodelling* is another factor. Once bones have grown the bone continues to be replaced on an ongoing basis and this can lead to a change in shape of the bone. Interestingly the opposite law applies here. High compressive stresses tend to stimulate the production of more bone whereas lower stresses suppress this. The third factor is that cartilaginous bone can actually be deformed mechanically and this may be particularly important in the feet where some bones are not fully calcified until around the age of 10 years.

A further common impairment is contracture of the joint capsule. This is particularly common at the knee but may also restrict extension and internal/external rotation of the hip. It results from contracture of the ligaments which form the joint capsule and is thus quite distinct from contracture of the muscle. It is included with bony deformities because the capsule is a deep structure and quite difficult to approach surgically. Management of joint contractures is thus often achieved through bony surgery similar to those used to manage bony malalignment.

Clinical management

Natural history

Establishing the natural history of cerebral palsy is now quite difficult because it is unethical to deprive children of the benefits of modern medicine. Children seen for gait analysis will typically have had delayed motor milestones such as the age at which they first sat, crawled or walked. Spasticity may be evident very early and weakness (particularly around the hips) is also common in early childhood but contracture and bony malalignment are less evident. These tend to develop in middle and late childhood. Although weakness can be a significant issue from quite early on, it becomes much more significant as children increase their bodyweight rapidly through adolescence.

Spasticity management

The focus of management in early childhood is generally on trying to reduce spasticity and a range of options are available. Although there are some anecdotal reports of responses to stem cell implants there is little scientific evidence so far that anything can be done to repair the original brain damage. *Botulinum toxin* is a chemical that disrupts the neuromuscular junction and thus prevents the neural input to a muscle activating it. If injected into the muscle it is selectively absorbed by these junctions and is an excellent way of suppressing activity in specific muscles. The direct effect of the toxin wears off over a period of between 3 and 9 months (Eames et al., 1999). This can be useful as it is possible to test the effects of injections without the risk of doing permanent harm but does mean that, if successful, injections need to be repeated. In children with cerebral palsy who can walk, the gastrocnemius muscles are the most commonly injected (Baker et al., 2002; Eames et al., 1999). In severe spasticity it may be more effective simply to release specific muscles surgically rather than perform repeat injections.

If spasticity affects many muscles then a specific intervention such as botulinum toxin is less appropriate. *Selective dorsal rhizotomy* (SDR) is surgery to the spine which cuts a proportion of the nerves in the dorsal roots typically in the lumbar and sacral spine. This reduces neural activity in the reflex arc and thus reduces spasticity in all muscles innervated from that level of the spine. The word selective in SDR refers to using electromyography (EMG) during the surgery to select the rootlets to cut and how many. SDR is only suitable for a small number of children and requires highly specialised surgical teams. Another approach is to use baclofen, which is an analogue of a naturally occurring inhibitory neurotransmitter and thus suppresses spasticity generally. It can be taken orally but little of it crosses the blood–brain barrier into the cerebrospinal fluid, therefore large doses are required. Another option is to surgically insert a pump that will deliver the drug directly into the intrathecal space of the spine and is known as intrathecal baclofen (ITB). ITB tends to be used only for more severely involved children (occasionally in GMFCS III but most commonly for GMFCS IV and V).

Muscle and tendon surgery

As children age, muscle contractures generally become more significant. As these are not a direct consequence of neural activity they will not be affected by any of the spasticity reduction techniques. A variety of surgical procedures performed on either muscle or tendon are thus required. Perhaps the most common is the gastrocnemius recession in which the tendon linking the muscle to the Achilles tendon is cut. This is also referred to as Achilles tendon lengthening or heel cord lengthening. Partial releases of muscles such as the hamstrings, psoas and hip adductor muscles can also be performed to allow for more normal gait and posture. If the rectus femoris is contracted it can be useful not just to release it but to transfer its insertion from the patella (where it acts as a knee extensor) to the posterior aspect of the proximal tibia (where it may act as a knee flexor). The longer tendons of the tibialis anterior and posterior can be divided longitudinally and part of the tendon can be transferred to the other side of the foot to provide a 'stirrup' that can stabilise the ankle and subtalar joint in the coronal plane.

Bony surgery

Femoral anteversion and tibial torsion are rotational deformities of the bone and can be corrected by surgical procedures such as cutting the bone transversely, untwisting the bone and attaching a metal plate by screws to hold the bone in this new alignment while it heals. External fixation may also be used to correct rotational deformities. Bony malalignment of the feet can be corrected by performing various osteotomies to the bones of the foot. The most common of these is the calcaneal lengthening in which the calcaneus is cut through and a bone graft placed in the gap to lengthen the bone and swing the foot internally.

Joint capsule contractures can also be improved by bony surgery. Thus severe knee capsule contractures can be corrected by taking a wedge out of the anterior aspect of the distal femur. Milder contractures can be managed by *guided growth*. In this, staples or eight plates are inserted across the anterior aspect of the distal femoral growth plate. This prevents the bone growing anteriorly and the growth that does occur posteriorly negates the effect of the capsular contracture. Placing staples anteriorly and posteriorly can prevent any longitudinal growth and can be useful to correct any leg-length discrepancy.

In the past surgeons tended to perform the different surgical procedures on different occasions. More recently and particularly as surgeons' confidence has grown there has been a tendency towards performing a range of different procedures, to bone and muscle, within the same operation. This is often known as *single event multi-level surgery (SEMLS)* acknowledging the intention that only one operation would be required.

Strengthening

Now that the importance of weakness in cerebral palsy has been acknowledged there has been considerable research into physiotherapy programmes to actively strengthen muscles (Damiano and Abel, 1998; Damiano et al., 1995, 2002; Dodd and Taylor, 2005; Dodd et al., 2002, 2003). These generally used the principles of progressive resistive strength training, which have now been demonstrated to result in increases in muscle strength in children with cerebral palsy of up to 25% (which is consistent with their use in many other conditions). Such programmes are now being used more and more routinely.

Gait analysis

Clinical gait analysis

The most obvious use of clinical gait analysis is for planning complex, multilevel orthopaedic surgery. In most cases the surgeon already knows that surgery is required, and the aim of the gait analysis is to determine exactly which combination of surgical procedures will be of most benefit to the individual child. Many centres will also perform follow-up analysis, often between 1 and 2 years after surgery to assess outcomes as part of clinical audit. This allows the clinical team to benefit from the experience in managing each child and is important to maintain and improve levels of service provision. Gait analysis can also be useful in planning botulinum toxin injections, physiotherapy, orthotic interventions and more general monitoring of progress. Unfortunately the cost, availability and time required for the analysis often precludes its use for routine clinical purposes.

We will now focus on how clinical gait analysis is able to support surgical decision making. Gait analysis is only part of this process which includes capturing gait data, performing a comprehensive physical examination and providing a biomechanical analysis of the results. The actual decision as to whether surgery is required and which procedures should be included requires consideration of a number of other issues such as medical imaging, patient's history and psychosocial background and the surgeon's competences and level of support, which are outside the scope of this book.

Clinical gait analysis works within a framework of clinical governance that ensures that the services delivered to patients are both safe and of the highest quality. This includes a commitment to evidence-based practice, which requires that all techniques used should be well established and have been the subject of rigorous research. This is different from gait analysis in an academic environment, where innovation and experimentation are encouraged.

Data capture

Most clinical services focus on obtaining good-quality kinematic and kinetic data based on the measured positions of retro-reflective markers using techniques documented elsewhere in this book. The conventional gait model (CGM) (Baker and Rodda, 2003; Davis et al., 1991; Kadaba et al., 1990; Ounpuu et al., 1996) is by far the best documented and most common approach (see Chapter 4). Other models are used but it is questionable whether they have yet been sufficiently well validated in clinical practice to satisfy the strict demands of clinical governance. Many centres will also capture EMG data either concurrently with full kinematic data or with a reduced marker set.

Children are generally asked to walk up and down in bare feet first and with the minimum walking aids to achieve a reasonable gait pattern. This information gives the best indication of what their body is capable of. They may then be asked to walk when wearing their ankle foot orthoses and any other usual walking aids to give an indication of how they usually walk. As well as capturing full three-dimensional gait analysis data, it is important to capture good-quality standardised video recordings of the child walking.

Clinical examination

In addition to the gait analysis, a full clinical examination is also completed. The range of movement of various joints is assessed which helps identify muscle and joint contractures. Muscle testing is generally carried out, grading muscles on the conventional five-point scale (Kendall and Kendall, 1949) and this is often accompanied by a simple assessment of the degree of selectivity with which the child can control muscle activation. The Tardieu test (Boyd and Graham, 1999) is used to measure spasticity and the modified Ashworth scale (Bohannon and Smith, 1987), while often referred to as a measure of spasticity, should probably be regarded as a measure of resting tone. Measures of bony malalignment such as femoral anteversion and tibial torsion are also recorded. An example of the results of such a clinical examination are included in Figure 6.3. The results of the clinical examination give additional information which aids the process of interpreting the gait analysis data to elucidate exactly which impairments are most affecting the gait pattern.

Interpretation

In the context of providing data on which to select appropriate procedures for multilevel surgery the aim of the interpretation is to list the impairments that the child has that are most affecting the walking pattern. This process can be thought of as having four stages: orientation, mark-up, grouping and reporting.

Orientation

The first thing the clinician must do is obtain a general impression of the child and how they are walking. This will require a knowledge of the diagnosis (assumed here to be cerebral palsy), motor type,

	Left	Right
Hip extension range (Thomas)	7° ext	8° ext
Hip flexor strength	5 (2)	5 (2)
Hip extensor strength (knee 0°)	5 (2)	5 (2)
Hip extensor strength (knee 90°)	5 (2)	5 (2)
Hip abduction range (hip 0°, knee 0°)	44° abd	53° abd
Hip abduction range (hip 0°, knee 90°)	NT	NT
Hip abductor strength	5 (2)	5 (2)
Hip internal rotation range	41° int	33° int
External rotation range	31° ext	42° ext

	Left	Right
Femoral anteversion	11° int	12° int

	Left	Right
Knee extension range (capsule)	5° hyp	10° hyp
Popliteal angle	27° flex	26° flex
True popliteal angle	20° flex	25° flex
Dynamic popliteal angle	43° flex	40° flex
Knee flexor strength	5 (2)	5 (2)
Knee extensor strength	5 (2)	5 (2)
Quadriceps lag	0° flex	0° flex
Duncan-Ely (slow)	none	none
Duncan-Ely (fast)	none	none

	Left	Right
Dorsiflexor strength	4 (2)	4 (2)
Confusion (+/−)	neg	neg
Dorsiflexion (knee 90°)	5° pf	4° df
Dorsiflexion (knee 0°)	5° pf	4° df
Plantarflexor spasticity (Tardieu)	10° pf	3° df
Plantarflexor tone (Ashworth)	0	0
Plantarflexor strength (knee 90°)	4 (2)	4 (2)
Invertor strength	5 (2)	5 (2)
Evertor strength	4+ (2)	4 (2)

	Left	Right
Tibial torsion	20° ext	13° ext

	Left	Right
Thigh-hindfoot angle	0°	2° ext
Hindfoot-forefoot angle	14° int	16° int
Ankle equinus/calcaneus	mild equinus	neutral
Hindfoot valgus/varus	neutral	mild varus
Planus/cavus	neutral	mild planus
Forefoot abd/add	mod add	mod add

Weight (kg)	31 kg	
Height (cm)	133 cm	
True leg length (cm)	69 cm	69 cm
Apparent leg length (cm)	75 cm	75 cm

Fig. 6.3 • Typical physical examination for clinical gait analysis. Range of motions measures are in the [____] boxes, muscle strength in the [____], neurological signs in [____] and bony or capsular deformities in [____].

GMFCS classification and topographical distribution. Scales indicating the child's general level of functions such as the Functional Assessment Questionnaire (Novacheck et al., 2000) or the Functional Mobility Scale (Harvey et al., 2007) may also be useful. It is also important to have an overview of the child's medical and surgical history and of the precise reason they have been referred for gait analysis. The final part of orientation is to look at the video to get an overall impression of the gait pattern. During the assessment the child or family should be asked whether the walking pattern adopted during the analysis is representative of the way they usually walk.

It is also necessary to get orientated to the data. Graphs with data from several walks over-plotted should be reviewed to understand how much variability the child has exhibited. If a representative trial is to be singled out for the definitive analysis then this should be checked to ensure it is representative of all walks. It is also necessary to assess the data (gait data and clinical examination) for any signs of measurement artefacts. Comparing kinematic data with the video is useful here. Video is two-dimensional and the three-dimensional data may be needed to explain what you are seeing but should not contradict it.

Mark-up

The next stage is to look at the data and identify *gait features*. These are regions of the traces that are different from reference data from a population that has

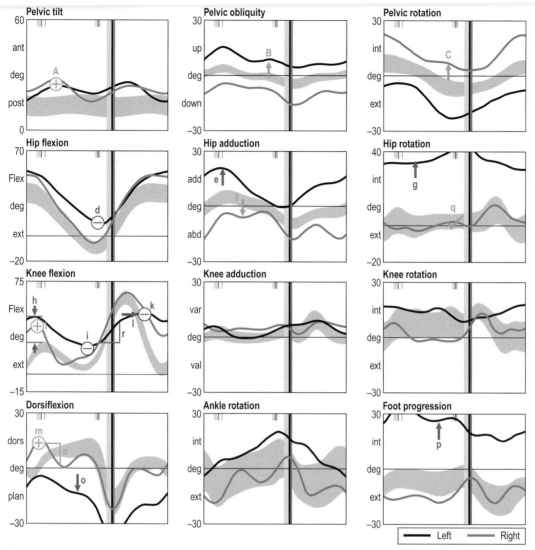

Fig. 6.4 • Representative graph marked up to identify features of the gait pattern.

no neuromusculoskeletal impairments. Many gait analysts do this in their head but it can be extremely useful to actually annotate the graphs to mark-up these features (Figure 6.4), using the symbols that are listed in Table 6.4.

Grouping

Once the gait features have been identified then the next stage of the process is to group the features that are thought to indicate the presence of a specific impairment and to relate these to relevant aspects of the clinical examination. It can be useful to list the evidence for a particular impairment as illustrated in Table 6.5.

Reporting

The final stage requires a report of the findings to be written to the referring clinician. If the process outlined above has been followed then this can be as simple as listing the impairments and including the evidence boxes and the marked-up gait traces in support of the analysis.

Conclusion

Gait analysis is now regarded as an essential component of planning surgery for children with cerebral palsy in many parts of the world. Very general gait

Table 6.4 Symbols for mark-up

Symbol	Meaning
$\ominus$	Too little (during particular phase in gait cycle)
$\oplus$	Too much (during particular phase in gait cycle)
↓	Too little (throughout gait cycle)
↑	Too much (throughout gait cycle)
↕	Increased range
⤓	Decreased range
▽ or △	Abnormal slope
→	Too late
←	Too early
↔	Increased duration
▶ ◀	Decreased duration
✓	Within normal limits
?	Possible artefact
⬭	Other feature (ring around feature)

Symbols are written on the charts in green for the right side, and black for the left side. Capital letters indicate bilateral features (including those of the pelvis).

patterns can be identified visually but gait analysis is important because every child is affected differently by the condition. Although it is caused by brain damage which directly affects the nervous system, children also develop muscle and joint contractures, bony malalignment and muscle weakness. There are now a number of different options for improving walking ability or preventing deterioration including spasticity management, orthotics, physiotherapy and orthopaedic surgery. It is in assessing children for complex surgery that gait analysis is most often used. When a surgeon requests gait analysis he or she is generally confident that surgery is required but needs to know which particular impairments are most affecting that individual child's walking. These can be identified by identifying features within the gait data and associating these with findings from the clinical examination.

Key points

- Cerebral palsy is caused by brain damage but this leads to a wide range of impairments including spasticity, weakness, muscle and joint contracture and bony malalignment.
- Common gait deviations during swing phase include equinus, excessive flexion of the knee and hip, and foot drop.
- Common gait deviations during stance include minimal to no heel contact and excessive hip and knee flexion.
- Each child with cerebral palsy has a distinct and unique gait pattern depending on their impairments and how they compensate for these.

Table 6.5 Lists some of the features and supplementary data identified in Figure 6.3 that suggest the child has femoral anteversion

Features	Comments		
g.	Too much left int. hip rot^n throughout cycle		
p.	Too much int. foot prog^n throughout cycle		
c.	Too much ext. rot^n of left pelvis throughout cycle Partial compensation for hip int. rot^n		

Supplementary data	Left	Right	Comments
Hip internal rotation range	50°	35°	
Hip external rotation range	0°	30°	
Femoral anteversion	30°	10°	From clinical exam

Impairment: **left femoral anteversion**
Evidence: **clear**
Effect on walking: **major**

- There are a wide range of options for improving walking ability and preventing deterioration including botulinum toxin, selective dorsal rhizotomy, intrathecal baclofen, physiotherapy, orthotics, strengthening programmes and orthopaedic surgery.
- Gait analysis may be used to plan complex orthopaedic surgery. The goal is to identify which impairments are having the largest effect on walking from features in the gait data and the clinical examination.

Gait assessment in stroke

Worldwide, 15 million people experience a stroke each year. Of these, 5 million experience permanent disability (WHO, 2010). Disability from stroke affects millions of individuals in the USA, with over 700 000 new cases annually. US statistics show that stroke is the third leading cause of death and the leading cause of serious long-term disability. Stroke management is estimated to cost the USA $68.2 billion annually (Centers for Disease Control and Prevention, 2010).

Gait dysfunction post-stroke is common, arising from the primary impairments associated with the neurologic event as well as from secondary cardiovascular and musculoskeletal consequences from disuse and physical inactivity. Muscle weakness, tone dysfunction, impaired motor control, decreased soft tissue flexibility and reduced cardiovascular function are major contributors (Carr and Shepherd, 2003). Regaining the ability to walk is the personal rehabilitation goal most frequently declared by persons post-stroke (Bohannon et al., 1988). Walking is considered important for return to independent living and full community access. Thus, whenever possible rehabilitation professionals provide gait examination and rehabilitation as part of post-stroke management.

Temporal and spatial parameters

Post-stroke gait is frequently characterised as slow and asymmetrical (Hesse et al., 1997; Olney and Richards, 1996; Roth et al., 1997; Woolley, 2001) with reduced cadence (Woolley, 2001) and there

is significant inter- and intra-subject variability (Olney and Richards, 1996; Woolley, 2001). Several authors suggest that hemiparetic gait deviations may be related to reduced gait speed (Carlsoo et al., 1974; Lehmann et al., 1987; Mizrahi et al., 1982; Roth et al., 1997; Wagenaar and Beek, 1992; Woolley, 2001). Roth and colleagues (1997) investigated the correlation between gait speed and 18 other temporal gait parameters for 25 people post-stroke. Since post-stroke gait speed was related to most, but not all, other temporal gait characteristics, the authors suggest that clinical gait examination must include gait speed with descriptions of asymmetry and paretic limb stance and swing phase durations and proportions. Many other spatiotemporal parameters frequently change post-stroke, including increased double support time, increased stance time by the non-paretic limb, shortened paretic limb step length, a moderately wider base of support, and slightly greater toe out angles (Carr and Shepherd, 2003; Montgomery, 1987; Olney and Richards, 1996; Perry, 1969; Shumway-Cook and Woollacott, 2007; Woolley, 2001).

Balasubramanian and colleagues (2009) explored temporal and spatial gait characteristics for an age-matched healthy control group and post-stroke groups of varying severity (severe, moderate, mild), step symmetry (longer, shorter, symmetrical) and fall risk (Dynamic Gait Index (DGI) ≤ 19 and DGI > 19). The authors confirmed increased variability in step length, swing, pre-swing and stride times during hemiparetic walking as compared with normal gait. For subjects post-stroke, paretic leg swing time variability was increased compared with the non-paretic limb during gait. Between-leg differences in variability for other spatiotemporal characteristics were revealed in the participants with the most impaired performance. Slower walkers (speed < 0.4 m/s) had significantly reduced step width variability as compared to age-matched controls. Patla et al. (2002) previously suggested that adaptation of step length, width, and height are important gait strategies employed by persons post-stroke to avoid obstacles and maintain balance. Balasubramanian and colleagues (2009) went on to explore gait characteristics' impact on function, by comparing gait characteristics across groups. They found that the post-stroke groups with increased step length variability and reduced step width variability also had poor performance outcomes (severe hemiparesis, asymmetric step and DGI ≤ 19). The authors ultimately suggest that the presence of decreased step width variability as well as increases in the variability of other gait parameters correlate strongly with impaired walking performance.

Kinematics

Common post-stroke gait deviations have been described (Brandstater et al., 1983; Burdett et al., 1988; Carr and Shepherd, 2003; Lehmann et al., 1987; Moore et al., 1993; Moseley et al., 1993; Olney and Richards, 1996; Pelissier et al., 1997; Perry, 1969; Shumway-Cook and Woollacott, 2007; Woolley, 2001).

For the paretic limb during stance phase these include:

- Decreased forward propulsion
- Forward flexion of the trunk with weak hip extension and/or hip flexion contracture notably contributing to a lack of hip extension in terminal stance
- Decreased or increased lateral pelvic displacement
- Poor hip position in hip adduction and/or flexion
- Trendelenburg limp caused by weak hip abductors
- Leg scissoring caused by spastic hip adductors and/or muscle substitution for weak hip flexors
- Excessive knee flexion in early and/or late stance
- Knee hyperextension during forward progression in mid-stance
- Equinovarus foot position with absent or inadequate heelstrike
- Varus foot
- Decreased dorsiflexion with mid-stance forward progression
- Inadequate ankle plantarflexion at toe off
- Unequal step lengths.

For the paretic limb during swing phase these include:

- Inadequate forward pelvic rotation
- Vaulting on non-paretic stance limb
- Inadequate and/or delayed hip flexion with abnormal substitutions such as hip circumduction, hip external rotation and/or adduction
- Exaggerated hip flexion
- Exaggerated trunk extension
- Inadequate knee flexion in early swing
- Delayed swing knee flexion
- Poorly controlled knee extension, particularly prior to heelstrike

- Persistent ankle/foot equinus or equinovarus
- Foot drop/toe drag or exaggerated dorsiflexion
- Excessive use of momentum resulting in an uncontrolled swing.

Moseley et al. (1993), Moore et al. (1993) and colleagues collectively hypothesise that both stance and swing phase gait deviations may be the result of an inability to selectively activate and coordinate muscle activity and/or maladaptive muscle shortening.

Olney and colleagues (1991) documented bilateral leg joint angles for individuals post-stroke walking at slow, medium and fast speeds. Joint angle amplitudes or joint ranges of motion differed from norms and present at all gait speeds. Considered clinically significant were the decreased amplitudes of knee flexion during swing and hip extension during stance for the paretic limb. A correlation between walking speed and maximum ankle plantarflexion on the non-paretic side was also documented. Hesse and colleagues (1997) first described significant differences in timing, step length, mediolateral displacement of the centre of pressure and centre of mass movement velocity patterns when persons post-stroke initiated gait with the affected versus the non-affected limb. Bensoussan et al. (2006) extended Hesse's work to assess the kinetic and kinematic gait initiation characteristics of three subjects post-stroke with spastic equinovarus foot and three control subjects. They observed that subjects post-stroke had asymmetrical movement strategies such as decreased support phase of the paretic limb when the non-paretic limb initiated gait; asymmetrical body weight distribution with the non-paretic limb accepting greater weight; more pronounced propulsive forces in the non-paretic versus the paretic limb; increased knee flexion during initial swing phase to accommodate for the equinovarus; and paretic limb flat foot initial contact.

Lu et al. (2010) studied gait during an 8 m walk and crossing obstacles of three different heights for both limbs for high-functioning individuals with chronic stroke (able to walk 100 m without an assistive device and Berg Balance Score >50). High-functioning individuals post-stroke had significantly different joint kinematics compared with an age-matched healthy control group, including greater leading toe clearance for clearing an obstacle, trailing toe obstacle distance, and posterior pelvic tilt regardless of leading limb. No significant differences were found for gait speed. The authors conclude that individuals post-stroke who are able to function at a high level develop a specific bilateral symmetrical strategy including increasing posterior pelvic tilt and elevating the swing toe. This strategy probably provides a more posterior placement of the trailing limb, increasing leading toe clearance during obstacle clearance, and preventing tripping.

Kinetics

Similar to gait spatiotemporal characteristics, force patterns post-stroke are described as highly variable between individuals as well as between paretic and non-paretic limbs (Carlsoo et al., 1974; Hesse et al., 1993; Marks and Hirschberg, 1958; Woolley, 2001; Wortis et al., 1951). Reduced vertical loading and significant variability of loading on initial contact has been documented for the paretic and non-paretic limbs post-stroke (Marks and Hirschberg, 1958; Wortis et al., 1951). Hesse and colleagues (1993) documented an increase in vertical loading after initial contact on the paretic limb as compared with the non-paretic limb as well as delayed loading after initial contact, premature unloading and reduced vertical push-off forces at terminal stance. Iida and Yamamuro (1987) reported significantly greater post-stroke medial-lateral centre of gravity displacement widths as compared with normal controls. They also described these differences to be more pronounced for individuals with more severe stroke.

Gait muscle activation patterns have been extensively studied in persons post-stroke. Well established is the high variability post-stroke in muscle firing magnitudes and phasic patterns between limbs and between individuals post-stroke (Carlsoo et al., 1974; Dimitrijevic et al., 1981; Peat et al., 1976; Richards and Knutsson, 1974; Takebe and Basmajian, 1976; Woolley, 2001). In a review of hemiplegic gait characteristics, Woolley (2001) concluded that the general muscular firing changes post-stroke include reduced magnitude for paretic limb muscles as well as premature onset and prolonged duration of firing across stance and swing phases for muscles in both limbs. Peat and colleagues (1976) reported a tendency for post-stroke paretic limb muscle activity to collectively peak at the same time after stance weight acceptance. A few studies have resulted in classification systems based on EMG patterns (Dimitrijevic et al., 1981; Knutsson and Richards, 1979; Waters et al., 1982), but none have gained broad translation for practical use in the clinic.

Nasciutti-Prudente and colleagues (2009) examined the relationships between muscular torque and gait speed in individuals post chronic stroke. They only identified one muscle group, paretic knee flexors, to have significant impact for predicting gait speed post-stroke. The paretic knee flexors accounted for 61% of the variation in gait speed, consistent with a previous study which identified paretic knee muscle strength as a moderate to strong predictor of walking ability in individuals post chronic mild to moderate stroke (Flansbjer et al., 2006).

It has been suggested that for the typical person post-stroke, walking requires approximately 50% to 67% more metabolic energy expenditure than that of a healthy person walking at the same speed (Corcoran et al., 1970) and that the paretic leg performs approximately 40% of the mechanical work of walking (Olney et al., 1991). Bowden and colleagues (2006) examined the effect of leg paresis on anterior-posterior ground reaction forces for individuals with varying levels of hemiparetic severity post-stroke. They documented a percentage of total propulsion generated by the paretic leg at 16% for severe hemiparesis, 36% for moderate hemiparesis and 49% for mild hemiparesis.

One clinical point of concern is the possible effect of gait compensation, such as hip hiking, vaulting, or knee hyperextension, on the non-paretic limb post-stroke. Kerrigan and colleagues (1999) estimated the non-paretic limb torques in all three planes about the hip, knee, and ankle for individuals with spastic paresis and stiff-legged gait post-stroke. They compared average stresses of the non-paretic leg with normal controls. In general, average peak non-paretic limb torque was not significantly different from that of controls, suggesting that the risk for biomechanical injury over time was minimal. This is counter to what clinicians might intuitively anticipate. More research is needed before clinicians may accurately anticipate the effects of long-term stroke compensation.

Clinical management

Already established in the rehabilitation community is the criterion of 1.1–1.5 m/s gait speed for safe pedestrian walking across different environmental and social contexts. Unfortunately only approximately 7% of patients post-stroke are discharged from rehabilitation able to walk 500 m continuously at a speed necessary for safe street crossing (Hill et al., 1997). Much more research is needed to establish best practices for regaining safe community-level gait.

Many persons post-stroke are either directed to or independently elect to use a unilateral assistive walking device. Kuan and colleagues (1999) studied the temporal and spatial gait characteristics of 15 subjects post acute stroke and nine age-matched healthy control subjects walking with and without a cane. They found that cane use had more of an effect on gait spatial variables than on temporal variables for subjects post-stroke. Gait phases remained similar regardless of cane use. For subjects post-stroke using a cane, the paretic side had increased pelvic obliquity, hip abduction and ankle eversion during terminal stance; increased hip extension, knee extension, and ankle plantarflexion during pre-swing; and increased hip adduction, knee flexion and ankle dorsiflexion during swing as compared with walking without the cane. The authors concluded that persons post-stroke may have improved spatial gait characteristics, including enhanced centre of mass translation and push-off in stance and decreased circumduction in swing, when using a cane.

Orthoses are also devices commonly considered for prescription post-stroke. Lewallen and colleagues (2010) documented gait characteristics for 13 individuals using an orthosis post-stroke, specifically solid, articulated and posterior leaf spring ankle foot orthoses. They found that gait was most impaired for those individuals wearing the solid ankle foot orthosis with a significant decrease in step length and gait speed. Use of the solid orthosis also resulted in slower decline walking compared with incline and walking over a level surface. Lehmann and colleagues (1987) reported a correlation between improved gait speed and ankle foot orthosis-related stance phase duration. A 5° dorsiflexed orthotic ankle angle contributed to increased walking speed and increase in heelstrike as compared with walking with no orthotic or when the orthotic was set in 5° of plantarflexion. The effect of a neutral ankle orthotic setting was not explored.

Also of interest to clinicians is the potential relevance of footwear choice to gait and balance for individuals post-stroke. Inadequate footwear has been identified as a fall risk factor for the elderly (Menz and Lord, 1999; Menz et al., 2006; Sherrington and Menz, 2003). While much more research is needed, footwear choice is probably important (Hesse et al., 1996; Ng et al., 2010). Ng and colleagues (2010) documented that a majority of their study participants preferred loose-fitting slippers for indoor walking over closed-fitting shoes and barefoot. Only 23% of participants reported that they had received advice about wearing appropriate footwear. The authors concluded that for proper ground contact, stability and proprioceptive input, it is reasonable to recommend shoes with broad flat heels, firm heel counter, thin firm mid-sole, laces or other fixation, and adequate slip resistance.

Key points

- Clinicians should expect high gait variability within and between patients post-stroke.
- Gait speed, using a standardised clinical protocol such as the 10 m walk, is an essential clinical measurement.
- To improve gait speed, knee flexion strength may be an important post-stroke measure as well as an intervention target.
- Gait intervention post-stroke must be individualised and based on the specific patient's demonstrated gait dysfunction.
- Intervention methods will likely involve improving flexibility, strength and task-specific ambulation activities.
- Gait training may incorporate both treadmill and over-ground walking, with specific attention to speed and safety within various functional environments.
- Environmental constraints must be considered when establishing goals for persons post-stroke.
- Devices, including canes, orthotics and footwear, are likely to impact gait characteristics on an individual basis. Exactly which gait characteristics change and to what extent, are yet to be determined. Gait analysis can be helpful to determine optimal use of these devices.

Gait assessment in Parkinson's disease

Parkinsonism is a disorder of the extrapyramidal system, caused by degeneration of the basal ganglia of the brain and is a common condition that affects motor function and gait. Parkinson's disease is a significant cause of morbidity with an estimated prevalence of 1.8% in those over 65 in Europe (de Rijk et al., 2000) with disease progression linked with a significant decline in quality of life (de Boer et al., 1996). The exact causal mechanism is not yet fully understood, however it is associated with a significant decrease in the number of dopaminergic neurons and an increase in the presence of Lewy bodies, tiny spherical protein deposits found in nerve cells whose presence in the brain disrupt the action of important chemical messengers. Diagnosis of Parkinson's disease is based on the presence of two or more of the following symptoms: tremor, rigidity, postural instability and akinesia. Akinesia is defined as a lack, or poverty of movement which can be subdivided into: slowness and unskilful movement secondary to rigidity, a lack or poverty of movement and difficulty in initiation of movement know as freezing.

Early analysis of gait in Parkinson's disease focused on temporal and spatial characteristics such as speed and step length, with Knutsson (1972) being one of the first to use gait analysis techniques to report the temporal and spatial parameters of gait in Parkinson's disease. Murray et al. (1978) conducted the first kinematic assessment of the gait of 44 men with parkinsonism using interrupted-light photography to record the displacement patterns of multiple body segments during free-speed and fast walking to quantitatively characterise their gait patterns and identified the following abnormalities:

1. Stride length and speed were very much reduced, although cycle time and cadence were usually normal
2. The walking base was slightly increased
3. The range of motion at the hip, knee and ankle were all decreased, mainly by a reduction in joint extension
4. The swinging of the arms was much reduced
5. The majority of patients rotated the trunk in phase with the pelvis, instead of twisting it in the opposite direction
6. The vertical trajectories of the head, heel and toe were all reduced, although others have commented on a distinct 'bobbing' motion of the head.

Parkinsonian gait is now widely recognised by a characteristic stooped and shuffling appearance (Samii et al., 2004). This includes a reduction in extension during late stance phase and a reduction in flexion during mid-swing coupled with a forwards inclination of the trunk (Fig. 6.5). The 'shuffling' gait occurs because the foot is still moving forward at the time of initial contact. In some patients initial contact is made by the flat foot; in others there is a heelstrike but with the foot being much more horizontal than usual. Some patients also show scuffing of the foot in mid-swing. Unlike most gait patterns, which stabilise within the first two or three steps, the gait of patients with parkinsonism often 'evolves' over the course of several strides. Figure 6.5 show steady state walking in an individual with Parkinson's disease compared with an age- and gender-matched normal subject.

Clinical management

One of the most well-validated treatments for Parkinsonism is L-DOPA which is a dietary precursor to dopamine. L-DOPA is converted to dopamine which improves the motor symptoms of rigidity and the ability to start and continue movements (bradykinesia) (Durrieu, 1998; Stowe et al., 2008; van Hilten et al., 2007). L-DOPA is recognised to have a short response (several hours) and a long response (several days or weeks) which both contribute to symptoms relief. Newly treated patients typically experience a 'honeymoon period' where the effects of L-DOPA help significantly, typically for several years. As time progresses this honeymoon period ends and the patient becomes more globally affected. As Parkinson's disease progresses patients experience motor fluctuations and other autonomic symptoms as the short response comes to an end (Morris et al., 2001), people with Parkinson's typically experience this as distinct *on* and *off* phases.

Morris et al. (1996) found that both gait speed and step length increased while on L-DOPA and although the gait parameters were repeatable when *on* medication they fluctuated greatly in the *off* phase of medication. O'Sullivan et al. (1998) found L-DOPA produced a significant increase in walking speed but not cadence, which again indicates that L-DOPA increases stride length, which was further confirmed by Defebvre et al. (2002). Ferrarin et al. (2004) used gait analysis to describe the inclination of the trunk and found a significantly reduced forward inclination or stooped gait pattern in Parkinson's disease patients on L-DOPA.

In addition to gait analysis clinical assessments are used. The Unified Parkinson's Disease Rating Scale (UPDRS) which is a validated scale for severity of Parkinson's disease, is commonly used (Box 6.1). The UPDRS has four components which have been largely derived from pre-existing scales. Parts II and III have the greatest relevance to gait analysis. Part II evaluates

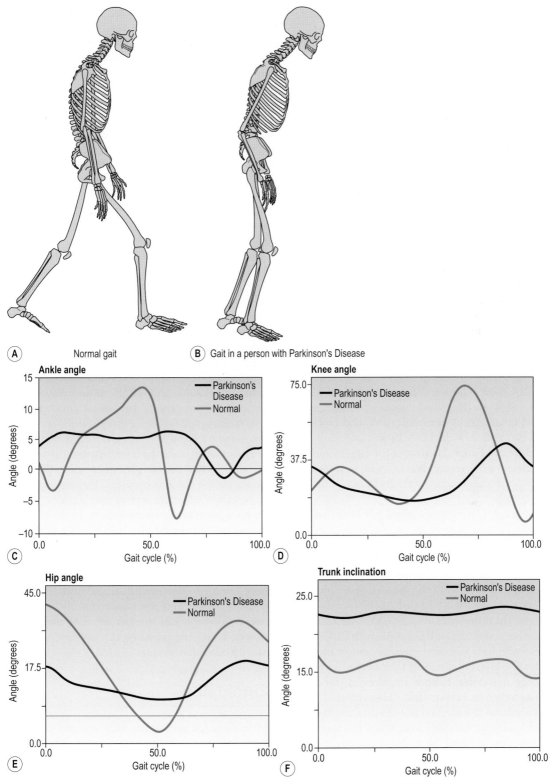

Fig. 6.5(A–F) • Ankle, knee, hip and trunk sagittal plane angles during gait in an individual with Parkinson's disease and an age matched normal individual.

The Unified Parkinson's Disease Rating Scale
- Part I: Mentation, behaviour and mood
- Part II: Activities of daily living
- Part III: Motor examination
- Part IV: Complications of therapy (in the past week)

activities of daily living in both the on and off phases which include falling, freezing when walking and walking. Part III is an assessment of motor capabilities and includes arising from a chair, posture, gait, postural stability, and body bradykinesia and hypokinesia.

Gait initiation problems in people with Parkinson's disease

Difficulties in initiation of movement known as freezing or motor blocks, remains one of the most debilitating aspects of Parkinson's disease (Halliday et al., 1998). Giladi et al. (1992) studied 990 people with Parkinson's disease and found 318 had motor blocks, 86% of these had blocks in initiation of gait, 45% had blocks in turning, 25% had blocks in doorways, and 23% had blocks in open runways. Therefore gait initiation affected the largest number of subjects with motor blocks, which accounted for 27% of the people with Parkinson's disease investigated.

Hass et al. (2005) investigated gait initiation and dynamic balance control in people with different severities of Parkinson's disease. They found that the peak magnitude of the centre of pressure (COP) to centre of mass (COM) distance was significantly greater during the end of the single-support phase in the less disabled patients than in more balance disabled patients. The differences in COP–COM distances between the groups suggest that people with Parkinson's disease who have impaired postural control produce shorter COM–COP distances than people without a clinically detectable balance impairment, which is an adaptation to prevent falls. Hass et al. (2005) concluded that this method of evaluation could prove a useful quantitative index to examine the impact of interventions designed to improve ambulation and balance in Parkinson's disease.

Jiang and Norman (2006) investigated the effects of visual and auditory cues on gait initiation in people with Parkinson's disease. Jiang and Norman found a mean difference in the maximum forward propulsive force between people with Parkinson's disease who freeze and do not freeze. Jiang and Norman also found a difference in the maximum horizontal force between the different cues. The auditory cues were rhythmic sounds with an interval matching the subject's average step time. The visual cues were high-contrast transverse lines on the floor adjusted for the subject's first step length and overall height. They found that transverse line visual cues improved gait initiation, while auditory cues had no effect. Although the use of high-contrast transverse lines on the floor can be applied to the home setting these are not readily available in the community setting.

Portable cueing aids aimed at helping people overcome difficulties in initiating walking or 'freezing' are becoming more common. McCandless et al. (2011) studied the effectiveness and acceptability of several of these devices on people with Parkinson's disease with gait initiation difficulties. Five randomised conditions were tested: laser cane, sound metronome, vibrating metronome, walking stick and uncued. Significant differences were seen in step length and COM and COP movement in the anterior/posterior and medial/lateral directions between freezing and non-freezing episodes. Significant improvements were seen in the COM and COP movement when using the laser cane and the walking stick and greater step length when using the laser cane during the freezing episodes. Participants rated the perceived effectiveness of the devices, which showed a significant improvement in satisfaction when using the laser cane for both starting and maintaining walking. Figure 6.6 shows the COM and COP patterns for uncued, cued using a laser cane and age- and gender-matched gait initiation. The cued condition improves the medial lateral movement of the COP and the anterior movement of the COM, however, there is still substantially less movement forwards when compared to the age- and gender-matched normal individual.

Conclusion

Gait analysis for both steady state gait and gait initiation is becoming more widely accepted as a sensitive tool for assessing Parkinson's disease. While general gait patterns can be identified, there is considerable variability of patients in particular when in the *off*

Paths of COM and COP during gait initiation

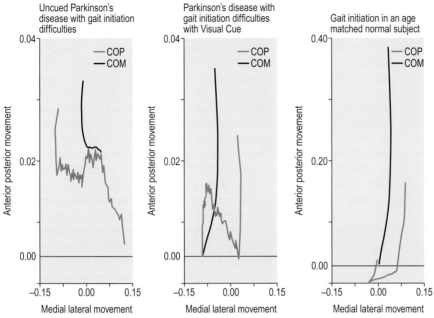

Fig. 6.6 • Centre of mass (COM) and centre of pressure (COP) movement.

treatment phase. However, the use of clinically based gait analysis is restricted to a small number of specialist clinics.

Key points

- Trunk inclination and hip flexion/extension are useful clinical outcome measures, however, temporal and spatial parameters are also good clinical markers.
- Clinicians should expect considerable gait variability between patients and between the *on* and *off* phases of the same patient.
- It is important to assess both steady-state gait and gait initiation in people with Parkinson's disease.
- L-DOPA improves the motor symptoms of rigidity and the ability to start and continue movements.
- Devices including walking aids and visual cues have been shown to improve gait characteristics and gait initiation. However, further work is required to determine the most effective devices in the community setting.

Gait assessment in muscular dystrophy

Muscular dystrophy (MD) describes a diagnostic subgrouping of progressive neuromuscular diseases resulting from genetically linked, non-inflammatory, myopathic disease. Duchenne muscular dystrophy (DMD), the most common paediatric-onset neuromuscular disease with an incidence of 1:3500–6000 males, leads to progressive deterioration of gait mechanics as the disease progresses (Bushby et al., 2010). The combined effect of weakness resulting from the death of healthy muscle tissue and the hypoextensibility caused by deposition of fatty and fibrous tissue within the muscle produce relatively predictable changes in posture and movement patterns of children with DMD during the first two decades of life (Rahbek et al., 2005).

Considerable variance has been documented in timing of onset and speed of progression of DMD, however the typical clinical presentation is a functional deterioration of movement capacity in the lower extremities usually presenting 2–3 years

143

before weakness in the upper extremities. This contributes significantly to the early compensatory patterns observed in children with DMD as they learn to accommodate for weaker muscle groups by modifying joint alignment and muscle firing patterns. Early in the disease progression, children with DMD will reduce their walking speed as a subtle means of altering gait kinematics to more easily advance the leg during swing phase and to reduce the energy expenditure of walking (Campbell et al., 2012; Perry and Burnfield, 2010). A classic motor adaptation strategy demonstrated by children with DMD is the Gower's sign, where the arms are used to push against the thigh to assist with hip extension upon rising from sitting (Campbell et al., 2012).

The insidious nature of onset of this disorder between 2 and 5 years of age combined with these compensatory movement patterns may contribute to delayed identification of the early impairments associated with DMD. Monitoring changes in muscle strength and range of motion over time are essential examination components to help distinguish age-related variances in typical development from the atypical developmental trajectory demonstrated by children with DMD. Goniometric measurements or analysis of functional movement patterns can provide relatively objective assessments of change in joint mobility across all ages. However, obtaining reliable objective strength measures in very young children can be challenging. In children older than 5 years of age, classic manual muscle testing (MMT) can generally be applied to obtain serial strength measures. In older children, an alternative method for measuring decline in strength of specific muscle groups over time to more precisely interpret altered gait mechanics is quantitative muscle testing (QMT). QMT measures isometric force production capacity by using a force gauge to directly assess contractile activity in a particular muscle group while ensuring constancy of muscle length, joint angle and velocity (Stuberg and Metcalf, 1988). In addition to the specialised equipment required, the child must also demonstrate qualities of cooperation, motivation, attention and understanding of instructions to support reliable application of the QMT.

The diagnosis of DMD is most often made between 2 and 5 years of age, with the lack of gait maturation being one of the early hallmark signs. Early gait pathomechanics coupled with reports of walking reluctance, increased clumsiness with frequent falls, laboured efforts required to come to stand (as compared with age-matched peers) and absent heelstrike are common early clinical presentations (Campbell et al., 2012). Sutherland et al. (1981) categorized gait disturbances of children with DMD into three groups: early, transitional and late ambulators. When examining the gait variables of 21 youngsters with DMD across these groups, these researchers identified three gait characteristics as predictors of disease progression with 91% accuracy: cadence, dorsiflexion in swing and anterior pelvic tilt. Apart from the positive Gower's sign, the most notable early gait changes include altered cadence, a slight increase in hip flexion during swing phase and a decreased ankle dorsiflexion with foot drop occurring as the cadence continues to decrease. Associated with these gait pattern changes, the ground reaction force passes anterior to the knee joint during early single limb support with muscle weakness, most notably in the quadriceps. When examining gait patterns of a relatively homogeneous group of 21 children with DMD with a mean age of 72 ± 8.2 months, D'Angelo et al. (2009) confirmed previously reported data demonstrating excessive anterior tilt of the pelvis and abnormal knee pattern loading response. Additionally, these researchers reported significantly lower stride length values, significantly higher step width values with higher flexion and abduction movement patterns used to advance the limb during swing phase as compared with age-matched peers. When examining the effects of gait velocity on gait patterns of an older cohort of children with DMD between 7 and 15 years of age, Gaudreault et al. (2010) reported higher cadence, shorter step length, a lower hip extension moment, a minimal or absent knee extension moment and reduced or absent dorsiflexion moment at heelstrike when compared with age- and gender-matched peers. Gaudreault et al. (2009) had previously examined the contribution of plantar flexion contractures during the gait of 11 children with a confirmed diagnosis of DMD with a mean age of 9.2 ± 2.6 and reported that increased net plantar flexion moments at the end of the lengthening phase of the plantar flexors and forward shift of the COP served to help the children ambulate independently despite significant weakness in extensor forces.

During the late stage of ambulation, children with DMD demonstrate a marked increase in work output associated with a marked exaggeration of gait pathomechanics. Functional compensation for the increasing weakness in the gluteus maximus muscle produces an exaggerated anterior pelvic tilt with associated restricted hip extension during stance phase. Inability to maintain pelvic alignment during stance phase due to gluteus medius muscle weakness results in a positive Trendelenburg's sign (where the non-weight-bearing hip drops during single leg stance) and emergence of Trendelenburg gait pattern characterised by lateral flexion of the trunk towards the weight-bearing side resulting in increased shoulder sway and widened base of support. These gait alterations make it possible for the child with DMD to maintain the force line behind the hip joint and in front of the knee joint throughout single-limb support, thereby helping to rely on deep joint structures to assist in the maintenance of upright stance as a compensation for increasing weakness in hip and knee extensor muscles.

Reliable prediction of cessation of independent ambulation is an important management consideration for individuals with DMD. Sienko-Thomas et al. (2010) suggested that the loss of knee flexion in loading response may be an indicator of impending loss of ambulation while Bakker et al. (2002) found that strength loss in hip extension and dorsiflexion are the primary predictors. Siegel (1986) found that when the combined lag angle of active antigravity hip extension in prone (starting with hip flexed to 90°) and active knee extension in sitting (starting with the knee flexed to 90°) exceeds 90°, loss of independent ambulation is likely to occur within a few months. Other reported clinical methods to identify impending cessation of independent ambulation include a manual muscle test (MMT) of below grade 3 for hip extensor or below grade 4 for ankle dorsiflexors (McDonald et al., 1995), reduction in lower extremity strength by greater than 50% and prolonged time to ascend four standard steps (Brooke et al., 1989).

Clinical management

Advances in medical and pharmaceutical management of children with DMD have resulted in a change of the natural history of the disease process with increasing numbers of the children diagnosed with DMD surviving to adulthood. Advances have included delayed cessation of ambulation, delayed development of contractures and reduced numbers of surgical corrections, reduced use of long leg orthotics, decreased incidence of scoliosis and corrective back alignment surgeries, delayed pulmonary function decline, and increased survival into early

adulthood. Moxley et al. (2010) reported an increase in mean survival to 30 years of age during the decade of the 2000s, with the potential for that age to further increase in the present decade. This represented an increase of almost 5 years between 1990 and 1999 as compared with 2000 and 2009. As preventive management of children with DMD becomes more precise, and as the survival likelihood continues to increase, it is important for clinicians to monitor gait pattern carefully for signs of impending degeneration.

To better understand the management needs of children with DMD across the lifespan, the International Standard of Care Committee for Congenital Muscular Dystrophy convened a 3-day workshop in Brussels, Belgium, in November 2009, to develop a consensus statement based on input from experts in the field and from families directly impacted by DMD (Wang et al., 2010). Management recommendations to meet the emerging needs of individuals with DMD across the lifespan drawn from the consensus statement on standard for care for congenital muscular dystrophies developed during that meeting include: coordinating transition of care from paediatric to adult services; identifying and planning for post-secondary educational and vocational needs; preparing patients to manage their own healthcare needs; supporting patients and families in making decisions regarding advance care directives; and advocating for services to meet independent living needs, aide services and healthcare coverage (Wang et al., 2010).

DMD is a representative example of multiple progressive neuromuscular disorders that result in altered gait characteristics. Understanding the underlying factors impacting gait pathomechanics in clients with muscular dystrophy provides essential information to support optimal quality of life and promote prolonged independent ambulation for these individuals.

Key points

- Quadriceps insufficiency is the key factor influencing compensatory postural adaptations of increased anterior pelvic tilt, restricted hip extension in stance and equinus posturing.
- Displacement of the weight-bearing force line anterior to the knee joint and posterior to the hip joint coupled with plantarflexion muscle

tightness helps support independent ambulation despite significantly reduced extensor force generation capacity.

- Timing of cessation of independent ambulation may be reliably predicted.

- Advances in medical management leading to increasing life expectancy warrants inclusion of transition services as children with DMD transition from paediatric to adult services.

References

Baker, R., Rodda, J., 2003. All you ever wanted to know about the conventional gait model but were afraid to ask (CD-ROM). Women and Children's Health, Melbourne.

Baker, R., Jasinski, M., Maciag-Tymecka, I., et al., 2002. Botulinum toxin treatment of spasticity in diplegic cerebral palsy: a randomized, double-blind, placebo-controlled, dose-ranging study. Dev. Med. Child Neurol. 44 (10), 666–675.

Bakker, J.P., de Groot, I.J., Beelen, A., et al., 2002. Predictive factors of cessation of ambulation in patients with Duchenne muscular dystrophy. Am. J. Phys. Med. Rehabil. 81, 906–912.

Balasubramanian, C.K., Neptune, R.R., Kautz, S.A., 2009. Variability in spatiotemporal step characteristics and its relationship to walking performance post-stroke. Gait Posture 29, 408–414.

Bensoussan, L., Mesure, S., Viton, J., et al., 2006. Kinematic and kinetic asymmetries in hemiplegic patients' gait initiation patterns. J. Rehabil. Med. 38, 281–294.

Bohannon, R.W., Smith, M.B., 1987. Interrater reliability of a modified Ashworth scale of muscle spasticity. Phys. Ther. 67 (2), 206–207.

Bohannon, R.W., Andrews, A.W., Smith, M.B., 1988. Rehabilitation goals of patients with hemiplegia. Int. J. Rehabil. Res. 11, 181–183.

Bowden, M.G., Balasbramanian, C.K., Neptune, R.R., et al., 2006. Anterior-posterior ground reaction forces as a measure of paretic leg contribution in hemiparetic walking. Stroke 37, 872–876.

Boyd, R.N., Graham, H.K., 1999. Objective measurement of clinical findings in the use of botulinum toxin type A for the management of children with cerebral palsy. Eur. J. Neurol. 45 (Suppl. 96), 10–14.

Brandstater, M.E., de Bruin, H., Gowland, C., et al., 1983. Hemiplegic gait: analysis of temporal variables. Arch. Phys. Med. Rehabil. 64, 583–587.

Brooke, M.H., Fenichel, G.M., Grigs, R.C., et al., 1989. Duchenne muscular dystrophy: patterns of clinical progression and clinical effects of supportive therapy. Neurology 39, 475–481.

Burdett, R.G., Borello-France, D., Blatchly, C., et al., 1988. Gait comparison of subjects with hemiplegia walking unbraced, with ankle-foot orthosis, and with Air-Stirrup Brace. Phys. Ther. 68, 1197–1203.

Bushby, K., Finkel, R., Birnkrant, D.J., et al., 2010. Diagnosis and management of Duchenne muscular dystrophy Part 1. Lancet Neurol. 9, 177–189.

Campbell, S.K., Palisano, R.J., Orlin, M.N., 2012. Physical Therapy for Children, fourth ed. WB Saunders/Elsevier, St. Louis, MO.

Carlsoo, S., Dahllof, A., Holm, J., 1974. Kinetic analysis of the gait in patients with hemiparesis and in patients with intermittent claudication. Scand. J. Rehabil. Med. 6, 166–179.

Carr, J.H., Shepherd, R.B., 2003. Stroke Rehabilitation: Guidelines for exercise and training to optimize motor skill. Elsevier, London.

Centers for Disease Control and Prevention, Stroke Fastats. Online: www.cdc.gov/nchs/fastats/stroke (accessed 9.12.10.).

Corcoran, P.J., Jebsen, R.H., Brengelman, G.L., et al., 1970. Effects of plastic and metal leg braces in speed and energy cost of hemiparetic ambulations. Arch. Phys. Med. Rehabil. 51, 69–77.

D'Angelo, M.G., Berti, M., Piccinini, L., et al., 2009. Gait pattern in muscular dystrophy. Gait Posture 29, 36–41.

Damiano, D.L., Abel, M.F., 1998. Functional outcomes of strength training in spastic cerebral palsy. Arch. Phys. Med. Rehabil. 79 (2), 119–125.

Damiano, D.L., Vaughan, C.L., Abel, M.F., 1995. Muscle response to heavy resistance exercise in children with spastic cerebral palsy. Dev. Med. Child Neurol. 37 (8), 731–739.

Damiano, D.L., Dodd, K., Taylor, N.F., 2002. Should we be testing and training muscle strength in cerebral palsy? Dev. Med. Child Neurol. 44 (1), 68–72.

Davis, R., Jameson, E.G., Davids, J.R., et al., 1991. A gait analysis data collection and reduction technique. Hum. Mov. Sci. 10, 575–587.

Day, S.M., Wu, Y.W., Strauss, D.J., et al., 2007. Change in ambulatory ability of adolescents and young adults with cerebral palsy. Dev. Med. Child Neurol. 49 (9), 647–653.

de Boer, A.G., Wijker, W., Speelman, J.D., et al., 1996. Quality of life in patients with Parkinson's disease: development of a questionnaire. J. Neurol. Neurosurg. Psychiatry 61 (1), 70–74.

de Rijk, M.C., Launer, L.I., Berger, K., et al., 2000. Prevalence of Parkinson's disease in Europe: A collaborative study of population-based cohorts. Neurology 54 (11), S21–S23.

Defebvre, L.J.P., Krystkowiak, P., Blatt, J.L., et al., 2002. Influence of pallidal stimulation and levodopa on gait and preparatory postural adjustments in Parkinson's disease. Mov. Disord. 17 (1), 76–83.

Dimitrijevic, M.R., Faganel, J., Sherwood, A.M., et al., 1981. Activation of paralysed leg flexors and extensors during gait in patients after stroke. Scand. J. Rehabil. Med. 13, 109–115.

Dobson, F., 2007. Classification of Gait Patterns in Children with Hemiplegic Cerebral Palsy. School of Physiotherapy, University of Melbourne, Melbourne.

Dobson, F., Morris, M.E., Baker, R., et al., 2006. Clinician agreement on gait pattern ratings in children with spastic hemiplegia. Dev. Med. Child Neurol. 48 (6), 429–435.

Dobson, F., Morris, M.E., Baker, R., et al., 2007. Gait classification in children with cerebral palsy: a systematic review. Gait Posture 25 (1), 140–152.

Dodd, K., Taylor, N., 2005. Strength Training for Young People with Cerebral Palsy. La Trobe University, Melbourne.

Dodd, K., Taylor, N., Damiano, D., 2002. A systematic review on the effectiveness of strength training programs for people with cerebral palsy. Arch. Phys. Med. Rehabil. 83, 1157–1164.

Dodd, K., Taylor, N., Graham, H., 2003. A randomized clinical trial of strength training in young people with cerebral palsy. Dev. Med. Child Neurol. 45, 652–657.

Durrieu, G., 1998. Early combination therapy with levodopa and dopamine agonist for preventing motor fluctuations in Parkinson's disease. Cochrane Database Syst. Rev 2, CD001311.

Eames, N.W.A., Baker, R., Hill, N., et al., 1999. The effect of botulinum toxin A on gastrocnemius length: magnitude and duration of response. Dev. Med. Child Neurol. 41 (4), 226–232.

Elder, G.C., Kirk, J., Stewart, G., et al., 2003. Contributing factors to muscle weakness in children with cerebral palsy. Dev. Med. Child Neurol. 45 (8), 542–550.

Ferrarin, M., Rizzone, M., Lopiano, L., et al., 2004. Effects of subthalamic nucleus stimulation and -dopa in trunk kinematics of patients with Parkinson's disease. Gait Posture 19 (2), 164–171.

Flansbjer, U., Downham, D., Lexell, J., 2006. Knee muscle strength, gait performance, and perceived participation after stroke. Arch. Phys. Med. Rehabil. 87, 974–980.

Foran, J.R., Steinman, S., Barash, I., et al., 2005. Structural and mechanical alterations in spastic skeletal muscle. Dev. Med. Child Neurol. 47 (10), 713–717.

Fry, N.R., Gough, M., McNee, A.E., et al., 2007. Changes in the volume and length of the medial gastrocnemius after surgical recession in children with spastic diplegic cerebral palsy. J. Pediatr. Orthop. 27 (7), 769–774.

Gage, J.R., Schwartz, M.H., Koop, S.E., et al., 2009. The Identification and Treatment of Gait Problems in Cerebral Palsy. Clinics in Developmental Medicine. Mac Keith Press, London.

Gaudreault, N., Gravel, D., Nadeau, S., 2009. Evaluation of plantar flexion contracture contribution during the gait of children with Duchenne muscular dystrophy. J. Electromyogr. Kinesiol. 19, 180–186.

Gaudreault, N., Gravel, D., Nadeau, S., et al., 2010. Gait patterns comparison of children with Duchenne muscular dystrophy to those of control subjects considering the effect of gait velocity. Gait Posture 32, 342–347.

Giladi, N., McMahon, D., Przedborski, S., et al., 1992. Motor blocks in Parkinson's disease. Neurology 42, 333–339.

Halliday, S.E., Winter, D.A., Frank, J.S., et al., 1998. The initiation of gait in young, elderly, and Parkinsons disease subjects. Gait Posture 8, 8–14.

Harvey, A., Graham, H.K., Morris, M.E., et al., 2007. The Functional Mobility Scale: ability to detect change following single event multilevel surgery. Dev. Med. Child Neurol. 49 (8), 603–607.

Hass, C., Waddell, D., Fleming, R., et al., 2005. Gait initiation and dynamic balance control in Parkinson's disease. Arch. Phys. Med. Rehabil. 86 (11), 2172–2176.

Hesse, S.A., Jahnke, M.T., Schreiner, C., et al., 1993. Gait symmetry and functional walking performance in hemiparetic patient prior to and after a 4-week rehabilitation programme. Gait Posture 1, 166–171.

Hesse, S., Luecke, D., Jahnke, M.T., et al., 1996. Gait function in spastic hemiparetic patients walking barefoot, with firm shoes and with ankle-foot orthosis. Int. J. Rehabil. Res. 19, 133–141.

Hesse, S., Reiter, F., Jhanke, M., et al., 1997. Asymmetry of gait initiation in hemiparetic stroke subjects. Arch. Phys. Med. Rehabil. 78, 719–724.

Hill, K., Ellis, P., Bernhardt, J., et al., 1997. Balance and mobility outcomes for stroke patients: A comprehensive audit. Aust. J. Physiother. 43, 173–180.

Hullin, M., Robb, J., Loudon, I., 1996. Gait patterns in children with hemiplegic spastic cerebral palsy. J. Pediatr. Orthop. 5, 247–251.

Iida, H., Yamamuro, T., 1987. Kinetic analysis of the center of gravity of the human body in normal and pathological gait. J. Biomech. 20, 987–995.

Jahnsen, R., Villien, L., Aamodt, G., et al., 2004. Locomotion skills in adults with cerebral palsy. Clin. Rehabil. 18, 309–316.

Jiang, Y., Norman, K.E., 2006. Effects of visual and auditory cues on gait initiation in people with Parkinson's disease. Clin. Rehabil. 20 (1), 36–45.

Kadaba, M.P., Ramakrishnan, H.K., Wootten, M.E., 1990. Measurement of lower extremity kinematics during level walking. J. Orthop. Res. 8 (3), 383–392.

Kendall, H., Kendall, F., 1949. Muscles Testing and Function. Lippincott Williams & Wilkins, Baltimore, MD.

Kerrigan, D.C., Frates, E.P., Rogan, S., et al., 1999. Spastic paretic stiff-legged gait: biomechanics of the unaffected limb. Am. J. Phys. Med. Rehabil. 78, 354–360.

Knutsson, E., 1972. An analysis of parkinsonian gait. Brain 95 (3), 475–486.

Knutsson, E., Richards, C., 1979. Different types of disturbed motor control in gait of hemiparetic patients. Brain 102, 405–430.

Kuan, T., Tsou, J., Fong-Chin, S., 1999. Hemiplegic gait of stroke patients: the effect of using a cane. Arch. Phys. Med. Rehabil. 80, 777–784.

Lance, J., 1980. Pathophysiology of spasticity and clinical experience with baclofen. In: Feldman, R., Young, R., Koella, W. (Eds.), Spasticity: Disordered Motor Control. Year Book Medical Publishers, Chicago, IL, pp. 485–495.

Lehmann, J.F., Condon, S.M., Price, R., et al., 1987. Gait abnormalities in hemiplegia: their correction by ankle-foot orthoses. Arch. Phys. Med. Rehabil. 68, 763–771.

Lewallen, J., Miedaner, J., Amyx, S., et al., 2010. Effect of three styles of custom ankle foot orthoses on the gait of stroke patients while walking on level and inclined surfaces. American

Academy of Orthotists and Prosthetists 22, 78–83.

Lu, T.W., Yen, H.C., Chen, H.L., et al., 2010. Symmetrical kinematic changes in higher function in older patients post-stroke during obstacle-crossing. Gait Posture 31, 511–516.

Marks, M., Hirschberg, G.G., 1958. Analysis of the hemiplegic gait. Ann. N. Y. Acad. Sci. 74, 59–77.

McCandless, P., Evans, B., Richards, J., et al., 2011. The effectiveness and acceptability of different cueing devices for people with Parkinsons disease and gait initiation difficulties. Physiotherapy 97 (Suppl. S1), eS772.

McDonald, C.M., Abresch, R.T., Carter, G.T., 1995. Profiles of neuromuscular diseases: Duchenne muscular dystrophy. Am. J. Phys. Med. Rehabil. 74 (Suppl.), 570–592.

Menz, H.B., Lord, S.R., 1999. Footwear and postural stability in older people. J. Am. Podiatr. Med. Assoc. 89, 346–357.

Menz, H.B., Morris, M.E., Lord, S.R., 2006. Footwear characteristics and risk of indoor and outdoor falls in older people. Gerontology 52, 174–180.

Mizrahi, J., Susak, Z., Heller, L., et al., 1982. Variation of time-distance parameters of the stride related to clinical gait improvement in hemiplegics. Scand. J. Rehabil. Med. 14, 133–140.

Montgomery, J., 1987. Assessment and treatment of locomotor deficits in stroke. In: Duncan, P., Badke, M.E. (Eds.), Stroke Rehabilitation: The Recovery of Motor Control. Mosby, St. Louis, MO.

Moore, S., Schurr, K., Wales, A., et al., 1993. Observation and analysis of hemiplegic gait: swing phase. Aust. J. Physiother. 39, 271–278.

Morris, M.E., Matyas, T.A., Iansek, R., et al., 1996. Temporal stability of gait in Parkinson's disease. Phys. Ther. 76 (7), 763–777.

Morris, M.E., Huxham, F., McGinley, J., et al., 2001. The biomechanics and motor control of gait in Parkinson disease. Clin. Biomech. (Bristol, Avon) 16 (6), 459–470.

Moseley, A., Wales, A., Herbert, R., et al., 1993. Observation and analysis of hemiplegic gait: stance phase. Aust. J. Physiother. 39, 259–267.

Moxley, R., Pandya, S., Ciafolnoi, E., et al., 2010. Change in natural history of Duchenne muscular dystrophy with long-term corticosteroid treatment: implications for management. J. Child Neurol. 25 (9), 1116–1129.

Murphy, K., Molnar, G., Lankasky, K., 1995. Medical and functional status of adults with cerebral palsy. Dev. Med. Child Neurol. 37, 1075–1084.

Murray, M.P., Sepic, S.B., Gardner, G. M., Downs, W.J., 1978. Walking patterns of men with parkinsonism. Am. J. Phys. Med. 57, 278–294.

Nasciutti-Prudente, C., Oliveira, F.G., Houri, S.F., et al., 2009. Relationships between muscular torque and gait speed in chronic hemiparetic subjects. Disabil. Rehabil. 31, 103–108.

Ng, H., McGinley, J.L., Jolley, D., et al., 2010. Effects of footwear on gait and balance in people recovering from stroke. Age Ageing 39, 507–510.

Novacheck, T.F., Stout, J.L., Tervo, R., 2000. Reliability and validity of the Gillette Functional Assessment Questionnaire as an outcome measure in children with walking disabilities. J. Pediatr. Orthop. 20 (1), 75–81.

O'Sullivan, J.D., Said, C.M., Dillon, L.C., et al., 1998. Gait analysis in patients with Parkinson's disease and motor fluctuations: Influence of levodopa and comparison with other measures of motor function. Mov. Disord. 13 (6), 900–906.

Olney, S.J., Richards, C., 1996. Hemiparetic gait following stroke. Part 1: Characteristics. Gait Posture 4, 136–148.

Olney, S.J., Griffin, M.P., Monga, T.N., et al., 1991. Work and power in gait of stroke patients. Arch. Phys. Med. Rehabil. 72, 309–314.

Ounpuu, O., Davis, R., Deluca, P., 1996. Joint kinetics: Methods, interpretation and treatment decision-making in children with cerebral palsy and myelomeningocele. Gait Posture 4, 62–78.

Palisano, R., Rosenbaum, P., Walter, S., 1997. Development and reliability of a system to classify gross motor function in children with cerebral palsy. Dev. Med. Child Neurol. 39 (4), 214–223.

Palisano, R.J., Hanna, S.E., Rosenbaum, P.L., et al., 2000. Validation of a model of gross motor function for children with cerebral palsy. Phys. Ther. 80 (10), 974–985.

Palisano, R.J., Rosenbaum, P., Bartlett, D., et al., 2008. Content validity of the expanded and revised Gross Motor Function Classification System. Dev. Med. Child Neurol. 50 (10), 744–750.

Patla, A.E., Niechwiej, E., Racco, V., et al., 2002. Understanding the roles of vision in the control of human locomotion. Exp. Brain Res. 142, 551–561.

Peat, M., Dubo, H.I.C., Winter, D.A., et al., 1976. Electromyographic analysis of gait: hemiplegic locomotion. Arch. Phys. Med. Rehabil. 57, 421–425.

Pelissier, J., Perennou, D., Laassel, E.M., 1997. Lab analysis of gait in hemiplegic adults: review of literature. Ann. Readapt. Med. Phys. 40, 297–313.

Perry, J., 1969. The mechanics of walking in hemiplegia. Clin. Orthop. Relat. Res. 63, 23–31.

Perry, J., Burnfield, J.M., 2010. Gait Analysis: Normal and Pathological Function, second ed. Slack Inc., Thorofare, NJ, p. 168.

Rahbek, J., Werge, B., Madsen, A., et al., 2005. Adult life with Duchenne muscular dystrophy: observations among an emerging and unforseen population. Pediatr. Rehabil. 8 (1), 17–28.

Richards, C., Knutsson, E., 1974. Evaluation of abnormal gait patterns by intermittent light photography and electromyography. Scand. J. Rehabil. Med. 3, 61–68.

Rodda, J.M., Graham, H.K., Carson, L., et al., 2004. Sagittal gait patterns in spastic diplegia. J. Bone Joint Surg. Br. 86 (2), 251–258.

Rosenbaum, P., Paneth, N., Leviton, A., et al., 2007. A report: The definition and classification of cerebral palsy, April 2006. Dev. Med. Child Neurol. 49 (Suppl. 2), 8–14.

Roth, E.J., Merbitz, C., Mroczek, K., et al., 1997. Hemiplegic gait relationships between walking speed and other temporal parameters. Am. J. Phys. Med. Rehabil. 76, 128–133.

Rozumalski, A., Schwartz, M.H., 2009. Crouch gait patterns defined using k-means cluster analysis are related to underlying clinical pathology. Gait Posture 30 (2), 155–160.

Samii, A., Nutt, J.G., Ransom, B.R., 2004. Parkinson's disease. Lancet 363 (9423), 1783–1793.

Sherrington, C., Menz, H.B., 2003. An evaluation of footwear worn at the time of fall-related hip fracture. Age Ageing 32, 310–314.

Shortland, A.P., Harris, C.A., Gough, M., et al., 2002. Architecture of the medial gastrocnemius in children with spastic diplegia. Dev. Med. Child Neurol. 44 (3), 158–163.

Shumway-Cook, A., Woollacott, M.H., 2007. Motor Control: Translating Research into Clinical Practice, third ed. Lippincott Williams & Wilkins, Philadelphia, PA, pp. 299–329.

Siegel, I.M., 1986. Muscle and its Diseases: An Outline Primer of Basic Science and Clinical Method. Year Book Medical Publisher, Chicago, IL.

Sienko-Thomas, S., Buckon, C.E., Nicorici, A., et al., 2010. Classification of the gait patterns of boys with Duchenne muscular dystrophy and their relation to function. J. Child Neurol. 25 (9), 1103–1109.

Stanley, F.J., Blair, E., Alberman, E., 2000. Cerebral Palsies: Epidemiology and Causal Pathways. Mac Keith Press, Cambridge.

Stowe, R., Ives, N., Clarke, C.E., et al., 2008. Dopamine agonist therapy

in early Parkinson's disease. Cochrane Database Syst. Rev. 2, CD006564.

Stuberg, W.A., Metcalf, W.K., 1988. Reliability of quantitative muscle testing in health children and in children with Duchenne muscular dystrophy using a hand-held dynamometer. Phys. Ther. 68 (6), 977–982.

Sutherland, D.H., Davids, J.R., 1993. Common gait abnormalities of the knee in cerebral palsy. Clin. Orthop. Relat. Res. 288, 139–147.

Sutherland, D.H., Olshen, R.A., Cooper, L., et al., 1981. The pathomechanics of gait in Duchenne muscular dystrophy. Dev. Med. Child Neurol. 23 (1), 3–22.

Takebe, K., Basmajian, J.V., 1976. Gait analysis in stroke patients to assess treatments of foot-drop. Arch. Phys. Med. Rehabil. 57, 305–310.

Thompson, N.S., Taylor, T.C., McCarthy, K.R., Cosgrove, A.P., Baker, R.J., 2002. Effect of a rigid ankle-foot orthosis on hamstring length in children with hemiplegia. Dev. Med. Child Neurol. 44 (1), 51–57.

van Hilten, J.J., Ramaker, C.C., Stowe, R., et al., 2007. Bromocriptine/levodopa combined versus levodopa alone for early

Parkinson's disease. Cochrane Database Syst. Rev 4, CD003634.

Wagenaar, R.C., Beek, W.J., 1992. Hemiplegic gait: a kinematic analysis using walking speed as a basis. J. Biomech. 25, 1007–1015.

Wang, C.H., Bonnemann, C.G., Rutkowski, A., et al., 2010. Consensus statement on standard of care for congenital muscular dystrophies. J. Child Neurol. 25 (12), 1559–1581.

Waters, R.L., Frazier, J., Garland, D.E., et al., 1982. Electromyographic analysis before and after operative treatment for hemiplegic equinus and equinovarus deformity. J. Bone Joint Surg. Am. 64, 284–288.

Wiley, M.E., Damiano, D.L., 1998. Lower-extremity strength profiles in spastic cerebral palsy. Dev. Med. Child Neurol. 40 (2), 100–107.

Winters Jr., T.F., Gage, J.R., Hicks, R., 1987. Gait patterns in spastic hemiplegia in children and young adults. J. Bone Joint Surg. Am. 69 (3), 437–441.

Woolley, S.M., 2001. Characteristics of gait in hemiplegia. Top. Stroke Rehabil. 7, 1–18.

Wortis, B.S., Marks, M., Hirschberg, G.G., et al., 1951. Gait analysis in hemiplegia. Trans. Am. Neurol. Assoc. 76, 181–183.

Further reading

Opheim, A., Jahnsen, R., Olsson, E., et al., 2009. Walking function, pain and fatigue in adults with cerebral palsy: A 7-year follow-up study. Dev. Med. Child Neurol. 51 (5), 381–388.

Gait analysis in musculoskeletal conditions, prosthetics and orthotics

7

Jeremiah Tate   Julie Bage   Jim Richards   David Levine
Douglas Daniels   Natalie Vanicek

The aim of this chapter is to provide examples of how gait analysis can be used to determine the severity of musculoskeletal conditions and the efficacy of conservative and surgical management. This chapter will consider several common conditions and their management.

1. Total hip replacement
2. Knee osteoarthritis
   a. Conservative management
   b. Surgical management
3. Amputee gait
4. Orthotic management

Total hip replacement

Total hip replacement (THR) is a common procedure to reduce pain and restore function in individuals with osteoarthritis of the hip. A total of 231,000 THR procedures were performed in the USA in 2006 (DeFrances et al., 2008). The majority of THR procedures (55%) were performed on individuals over the age of 65, while 40% of THR procedures were performed on individuals between the ages of 45 and 64 (DeFrances et al., 2008). The incidence of primary THR is projected to increase 174% to 572,000 by 2030, and THR revisions to increase 137% to 96,700 annually (Kurtz et al., 2007).

It is important that rehabilitation professionals understand the resultant gait abnormalities following THR. The majority of studies have been conducted 6–18 months postoperatively and have concluded that gait does not return to normal following THR. In support of these studies, a recent meta-analysis demonstrated that physical function along with walking speed only returned to approximately 80% at 6–8 months postoperatively compared with normal subjects (Vissers et al., 2011) and some research suggests that abnormal gait patterns may contribute to the implant loosening (Foucher et al., 2009).

Spatiotemporal factors

Several studies have reported significantly decreased gait speed, cadence, step length and stride length at 1 month (Nankaku et al., 2007), 1 year (Perron et al., 2000; Tanaka et al., 2010), and 10 years (Bennett et al., 2008) postoperatively. Although 1 month postoperatively may be too early to identify persistent gait deviations, Bennett et al. (2008) provided strong evidence that spatiotemporal parameters may never return to normal. Conversely Miki et al. (2004) and Nantel et al. (2009) reported that gait speed had returned to that of normal controls at 6 months and 1 year postoperatively. However, the mean ages in these studies were 49 and 52.6 years, respectively, which is younger than usual candidates for THR.

Kinematics

Several studies have observed decreased motion in the sagittal plane about the involved hip, attributing this decrease in range of motion primarily to decreased peak hip extension prior to push-off (Fig. 7.1)

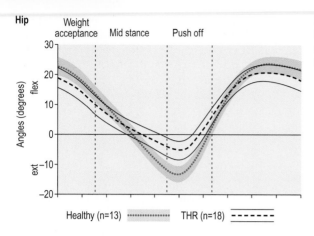

Fig. 7.1 • Demonstrating decreased sagittal plane hip range of motion, mostly the result of decreased hip extension during the late stages of stance (from Perron et al., 2000).

when compared with age-matched, healthy controls (Beaulieu et al., 2010; Bennett et al., 2008; Foucher et al., 2007; Perron et al., 2000). Bennett et al. (2008) and Perron et al. (2000) suggested that failure to fully extend the hip during late stance was correlated to decreased gait speed. Several studies have suggested that this decrease in hip extension may be linked to passive resistance or contracture in anterior hip structures (e.g., hip flexors) rather than hip extensor weakness (Miki et al., 2004; Nantel et al., 2009; Perron et al., 2000).

A significant increase in ipsilateral trunk lateral bending has also been observed during single limb support on the operated limb (Nankaku et al., 2007; Perron et al., 2000) along with decreased peak hip adduction angle (Beaulieu et al., 2010; Perron et al., 2000) when compared with age-matched, healthy controls. Both deviations are considered strategies to decrease demand on the hip abductors, to stabilise the pelvis in the frontal plane during single limb stance, by moving the centre of mass closer to the axis of rotation (i.e. the hip). Nankaku et al. (2007) concluded that lateral trunk bending led to increased energy expenditures. Beaulieu et al. (2010) also suggest that lateral trunk bending may be an attempt to improve balance.

Kinetics

Coupled with the changes in kinematics several changes in kinetics have also been identified. Perron et al. (2000) and Miki et al. (2004) observed a decreased internal hip extension moment during loading response, between 0 and 20% of the gait cycle, which correlated to the decrease in walking speed.

This is consistent with the kinematic findings of decreased hip extension range of motion influencing gait speed, suggesting that hip extensor strength is an important factor in the return to a normal gait pattern. In addition, a decreased internal hip abduction moment during mid-stance also occurred, which suggests weakness in the hip abductors (Beaulieu et al., 2010; Foucher et al., 2007; Perron et al., 2000). However, it has not yet been confirmed whether this hip abductor weakness is due to disuse atrophy from pain avoidance strategies prior to surgery, or the effect of the surgery. The lateral surgical approach to THR does involve the detachment and repair of the gluteus medius, yet many of the subjects studied underwent the procedure using a posterior approach, which leaves the abductors intact (Beaulieu et al., 2010). Hip prosthesis are in a greater degree of valgus than the natural femur, to reduce the bending moment. This puts the hip abductors at a mechanical disadvantage. Studies have also noted a decreased hip external rotation moment which may also be attributed to hip abductor weakness (Beaulieu et al., 2010; Foucher et al., 2009; Perron et al., 2000). This moment was identified as a significant determinant of peak implant twisting moment, which is critical for implant stability (Foucher et al., 2009).

Additional clinical relevance

Considering the longevity of the abnormal gait pattern and hip impairments a re-evaluation of current rehabilitation programmes of 2–3 months is warranted (Nantel et al., 2009). It has been suggested that long-term follow-ups (i.e. 6 months or 1 year) be performed with a goal of restoring normal gait pattern. Restoration of normal gait may help in preventing falls and reducing the risk of injury in more challenging activities (Nantel et al., 2009). Early and long-term intervention should focus on alleviating hip flexor tightness and strengthening of the hip extensors and abductors. Gait retraining may also be helpful in achieving a symmetrical and normal gait pattern, and potentially improve overall outcomes.

Key points

- A large increase in primary THR and THR revisions is expected over the next 20 years.
- The majority of studies indicate that gait does not normalise following THR.
- Rehabilitation should focus on improving hip extension flexibility, hip extensor and abductor strength, and symmetry of gait.
- Researchers suggest more long-term follow-up (i.e. 6 months or longer) to address persistent hip range of motion and strength deficits in efforts to normalise gait, decrease stresses on the implants and restore overall function.

Gait analysis in knee osteoarthritis

Peat et al. (2001) reported in an average population over the age of 55 years that 25% might have knee pain, with approximately 50% of these patients presenting with radiographic knee osteoarthritis. Knee osteoarthritis affects the medial compartment far more than the lateral compartment of the knee joint with an estimated 10:1 ratio between the occurrence of medial compartment to lateral compartment of the knee. This has been attributed to the mechanics of the knee in the coronal plane which shows between 60% and 80% of total load acting on the medial compartment during normal gait (Andriacchi, 1994; Baliunas et al., 2002; Hurwitz et al., 2002), and up to 100% of the load acting on the medial compartment in subjects with medial compartment knee osteoarthritis (Schipplein and Andriacchi, 1991).

The load distribution between the medial and lateral compartments is to be expected since medial compartment knee osteoarthritis is closely associated with a knee varus deformity, which gives rise to an external adduction moment at the knee throughout stance phase. The knee adduction moment is the product of the ground reaction force passing medial to the knee joint centre of rotation in the coronal plane. The knee adduction moment has therefore been used in many gait studies of knee osteoarthritis as an indirect measure of medial joint loading (Goh et al., 1993; Prodromos et al., 1985).

In a comparison of normal and medial compartment knee osteoarthritis adduction moments, Kim et al. (2004) found a significant difference in the adduction moment between the osteoarthritis group and an age- and gender-matched normal group, with the medial compartment knee osteoarthritis group having on average a 50% increase in their adduction moments (Fig. 7.2). Kim et al. (2004) also found a correlation between an increase in pain and decrease in function with an increase in knee adduction moment. Whether the knee starts in a varus position which leads to the adduction moment, which will then exacerbate the varus deformity, or whether the presence of an adduction moment causes the varus deformity is unclear. However, the importance of the varus deformity and knee adduction moment in the mechanics of medial compartment knee osteoarthritis is clear (Andriacchi, 1994; Crenshaw et al., 2000; Hurwitz et al., 1998).

Surgical management

There are several surgical approaches to the management of medial compartment knee osteoarthritis. These include total knee arthroplasty (TKA) replacement, uni-compartment knee replacement and high tibial osteotomy (HTO). The aim of all these methods is to reduce excessive loading on the medial compartment of the knee by correcting varus deformity, thereby reducing pain and improving function. In all surgical procedures the focus is on obtaining the best possible anatomical realignment of the pathological joint, which in turn aims to reduce the knee adduction moments to that of a pain- and pathology-free knee.

Total knee arthroplasty

Large numbers of TKAs are performed worldwide with 71,527 performed in England and Wales in 2008 (National Joint Registry for England and

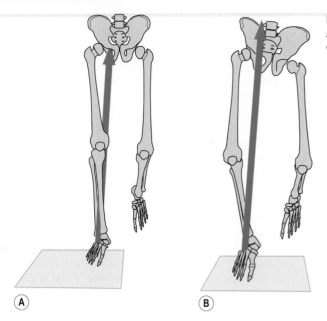

Fig. 7.2 • Knee adduction moments in (A) a pain- and pathology-free individual, and (B) an individual with medial compartment knee osteoarthritis.

(A)　　　(B)

Wales, 2009), with the prevalence expected to increase dramatically between 2005 and 2030 (Kurtz et al. (2007) with a projected 3.48 million TKAs performed annually in 2030 in the USA). The goals of the surgery are to alleviate pain, and restore alignment, stability and range of motion of the knee to improve patients' quality of life (Ranawat et al., 2005).

These patients typically undergo several weeks to months of rehabilitation following the procedure, thus it is highly important for rehabilitation professionals to understand the implications the surgery has on function. Specific to gait, research has demonstrated that TKA causes changes in both kinematic and kinetic parameters. Most studies have been conducted on patients in the long-term stages of recovery, defined as greater than 6 months postoperatively.

Kinematics

There have been multiple systematic reviews on the kinematics of the knee joint after total knee replacement. There is consistency among the literature that total (overall) knee range of motion is decreased in comparison to controls, with a reduction in the knee flexion during loading response (Milner, 2009) (Fig. 7.3). One systematic review found a range of 9.8–16.0° of knee flexion during the loading response for TKA patients versus 16.0–19.7° for controls (Milner, 2009). The same review found absolute differences of 3.0–11.2° in the range of motion between

loading response and peak knee flexion during stance. Additionally, TKA patients often demonstrate reduced knee flexion during swing and usually have a greater knee angle at heelstrike (McClelland et al., 2007; Milner, 2009).

Kinetics

Kinetic changes at the knee joint have been measured after TKA, particularly in the sagittal plane. In normal subjects, a biphasic moment pattern occurs during the stance phase of gait. An external moment across the knee, which causes extension, rapidly changes to a flexion moment, and then changes again to extend the knee and then flex the knee towards the end of stance (McClelland et al., 2007). Internal moments are generated by the leg musculature to counteract these external moments.

After TKA, this normal biphasic pattern is typically not present (McClelland et al., 2007). Depending on the alignment of the lower limb, a flexion moment or an extension moment may be present throughout the duration of stance. When an external flexion moment is present throughout stance, the quadriceps must generate the internal moment to a greater extent. This is termed the quadriceps overuse pattern. When an external extension moment is present throughout stance, there is an absence of quadriceps activity. This is termed the quadriceps avoidance pattern, which is typically discussed with regard to anterior cruciate

Fig. 7.3 • Knee flexion excursion from footstrike to peak knee flexion during weight acceptance in total knee arthroplasty and control groups across studies. With kind permission from Springer Science and Business Media.

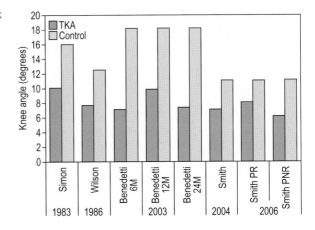

PR = Patellar Resurfacing   PNR = Without Patellar Resurfacing

ligament function (Timoney et al., 1993). Both patterns are common in the TKA population (Fig. 7.4) (McClelland et al., 2007).

The quadriceps avoidance pattern is clinically important as the hip or the ankle must compensate for the reduced knee extensor moment. Resultantly, studies have demonstrated that the hip extensor moment is typically increased in TKA patients compared with controls (Mandeville et al., 2007).

Additional clinical relevance

Quadriceps strength has been correlated with functional performance at both 3 and 12 months postoperatively. Yoshida et al. (2008) found that improved quadriceps strength resulted in significantly faster times in the timed up and go test, stair climbing test and 6-minute walk test ($p < 0.05$).

The available extension range of motion has been found to be a determinant of limb dominance during stance and walking. Harato et al. (2010) compared weight-bearing strategies of individuals with a diagnosis of bilateral arthritis that had undergone unilateral TKAs. Their findings suggest that patients who have sufficient extension range of movement (ROM) during stance utilise the operated lower extremity as the dominant side. However, patients with decreased extension ROM bear more weight on the contralateral limb, which could increase its rate of degeneration (Harato et al., 2010). One factor that could alter kinetics after TKA is patient weight, as compressive forces at the knee joint increase linearly with patient weight gain. One study found significant weight gain was common in the 2 years after total knee replacement. Specifically, 70 of 106 patients who had undergone a TKA gained an average of 6.4 kg (Zeni and Snyder-Mackler, 2010).

Mauer et al. (2005) compared the abilities of healthy age-matched controls to patients with bilateral TKAs in obstacle avoidance. The TKA group success rate in avoiding a suddenly appearing light band flashed on the floor was 30% less than controls. Clearly, this could lead to significant increases in fall risk and might be addressed in rehabilitation (Mauer et al., 2005).

High tibial osteotomy

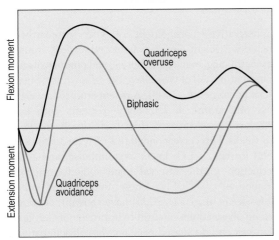

Fig. 7.4 • Quadriceps avoidance and overuse patterns (McClellan et al., 2007).

High tibial osteotomy (HTO) is another surgical procedure to alter the bony alignment and reduce the varus angle of the knee joint. The aim of an HTO

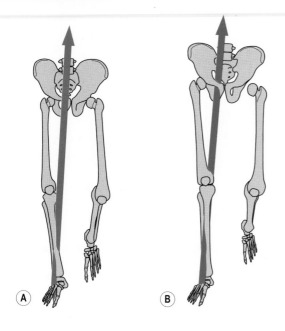

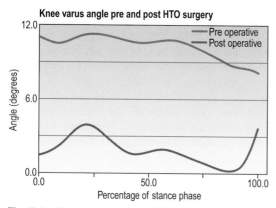

Fig. 7.5 • Pre- and post-high tibial osteotomy.

young. Prodromos et al. (1985) investigated the variable clinical results following HTOs for osteoarthritis of the knee with a varus deformity. They found that clinical success or failure could be predicted by the preoperative measurement of the coronal plane knee adduction moment, those patients with a high moment having a significantly worse result, with a recurrence of deformity, than those with a low moment. Briem et al. (2007) studied the effects of the amount of valgus correction using HTO for medial compartment knee osteoarthritis. Their results showed that physical function improved significantly overall. However, those subjects whose knee alignment was further away from the group's postoperative mean tended to improve less than those closer to the mean and have higher adduction moments 1 year after surgery. This again illustrates the importance of correct alignment during surgery and its relevance to adduction moments and clinical outcome scores.

As well as its use in comparative trials between two or more forms of treatment, gait analysis is also commonly used simply to quantify the benefit that a patient receives from a particular type of treatment. In such cases, a comparison may be made with pretreatment data values for that patient and with comparable results from normal individuals. Figure 7.5 shows an example of how the operation of HTO was successful in reducing the external adduction moment at the knee, and changing the varus alignment at the knee from 11° to 1.5°.

Conservative management of knee osteoarthritis

Conservative management of knee osteoarthritis includes weight loss, patient education, muscle strengthening, bracing (orthotics) and pharmacological intervention. All of these have been shown to be beneficial (Zhang et al., 2008). A recent study of a weight-loss programme in 157 obese patients with knee osteoarthritis decreased their body weight 13.5% in 16 weeks. This corresponded to a 7% reduction in knee joint loading, a 13% lower axial impulse, and a 12% reduction in the internal knee abductor moment (Aaboe et al., 2011). These findings and others (Messier et al., 2000, 2005) have shown that weight loss in obese adults can lead to improvements in function/gait and decreased pain and disability in patients with knee osteoarthritis. In addition, both patient

is to evenly share the load between the medial and lateral compartments of the knee. There are two main types of osteotomy for knee osteoarthritis, an opening wedge and a closing wedge. In an opening wedge, a cut is made in the tibia and the two sides are separated. The wedge-shaped space is filled with a bone graft. In a closing wedge, two cuts are made and a wedge-shaped piece of bone is removed. The two edges are then brought together creating the desired change angle. Both types of operation then require the bone to be fixed, usually with a plate and screws. HTOs are often seen as a way of delaying a total knee replacement in those considered too education and muscle strengthening have been found to have positive effects on knee osteoarthritis in improving function, including gait (Zhang et al., 2008).

Orthotic management of knee osteoarthritis has been studied in terms of improvements in joint forces during gait. Knee braces (direct orthotic management) and wedged insoles (indirect orthotic management) are becoming popular approaches in the management of medial compartment osteoarthritis. Both methods aim to influence the external forces applied to the knee, either by directly applying a system of forces or indirectly changing the ground reaction force.

The aims of knee valgus braces are to unload the painful compartment, through bending moments applied proximally and distally to the knee joint, and reducing the varus deformity (Pollo, 1998). Several studies have been conducted into the use of valgus knee braces for medial compartment osteoarthritis, and have reported that patients experience significant pain relief and an improvement in physical function (Hewett et al., 1998; Kirkley et al., 1999; Lindenfeld et al., 1997; Matsumo et al., 1997; Richards et al., 2005) and also a reduction in medial compartment load (Jones et al., 2006; Pollo et al., 2002). The use of valgus bracing in the management of knee osteoarthritis has been a point of debate for some time. Two of the most important biomechanical outcomes measures are the varus angle and the knee adduction moment during loading response. Bracing has been shown to reduce the degree the varus deformity by 3° and reduce the knee adduction moment by 14.5%, providing significant pain relief (Jones et al., 2006).

Another treatment that has been suggested is the use of lateral wedging of the foot. A lateral wedged insole has a thicker lateral border and applies a valgus moment to the heel, attempting to move it into an everted position. Lateral wedging has been found to significantly reduce the peak knee adduction moment during early stance and reduce pain (Butler et al., 2007; Jones et al., 2006; Keating et al., 1993; Shimada et al, 2006; Toda et al., 2001), however, Kakihana et al. (2007) found some inconsistency in knee varus moment reduction caused by a lateral wedging in knee osteoarthritis in approximately 18% of patients tested.

Research into the use of both knee braces and wedged insoles has shown positive clinical benefits and biomechanical benefits, which include a reduction in the knee adduction moment and varus angle of the knee joint.

Key points

- The prevalence of TKA surgery is expected to increase dramatically from 2005 to 2030 (Kurtz et al., 2007).
- TKA patients walk with less total knee ROM than age-matched controls.
- Gait abnormalities in the TKA population can result in either quadriceps under-activity or over-activity.
- HTOs are becoming a popular surgical intervention, however the correct alignment during surgery is very important to achieve the best clinical outcome.
- Improved quadriceps strength has been correlated with improved functional performance.
- Both conservative and surgical procedures can achieve anatomical realignment of the pathological joint and a reduction in the knee adduction moment.

Prosthetics and orthotics

Gait analysis can be of great value in the disciplines of prosthetics and orthotics. The alignment and adjustment of prosthetic limbs may be improved using objective measurements of gait, particularly if repeat trials are performed with different adjustments. The prescription of orthoses may be improved if the gait is monitored with the patient wearing different types or configurations of orthosis, for example with different ankle alignments on an ankle-foot orthosis for drop foot (Lehmann et al., 1987). Trials of different orthoses may also form part of the process of hypothesis testing, described above (Õunpuu et al., 1996).

The design and prescription of orthoses tend to be much more an art than a science and regrettably a significant proportion of orthotic devices are not used by the patients for whom they are made. Gait analysis is able to provide an insight into the functioning of orthoses and to compare different designs. It may also permit improvements to be made to existing designs, such as the Saltiel anterior floor reaction orthosis (Harrington et al., 1984). Some objective studies of orthoses have failed to demonstrate that they have any significant mechanical effects. It then becomes arguable whether the devices really do have no effect, or whether their mode of action is too subtle for the methods of measurement being used.

Gait analysis can also be used for the assessment of new or modified forms of lower limb prosthesis. It may be used to examine the effects of changing the design of a prosthetic limb, such as by altering the mass distribution (Tashman et al., 1985), or using knee joints with different types of braking mechanisms (Hicks et al., 1985). Two types of measurement are of particular value in this type of assessment: the kinematics of motion and the muscle moments and powers the amputee has to produce in order to be able to walk.

Measurement of the power output across the ankle joint is very valuable when comparing different prosthetic foot mechanisms. One of the major differences between the prosthetic foot and the natural foot is the inability of the prosthetic foot to generate power during pre-swing (third rocker). However, it is able to store energy during the second rocker and to release it during the third rocker, which may lead to a more natural gait pattern. Gait analysis can be used to examine the energy storage and recovery by prosthetic foot mechanisms and to determine how well particular types of foot suit different categories of patient. For example, a young subject who has had a traumatic amputation is much better able to take advantage of an energy-storing foot mechanism than an elderly subject who has received an amputation for vascular disease.

Amputee gait

An amputation is the surgical removal of a body extremity and results in the loss of the limb, and its associated skeletal structure, muscle function and proprioception. The majority of amputations occur in the lower limbs and at various levels: above the knee (transfemoral), below the knee (transtibial) and through the knee, ankle (Syme's disease) or forefoot. Bilateral amputations are less common. The primary causes are related to vascular disease, trauma and infection. The level of disability, discomfort and adaptations a person experiences following surgery vary according to the type of amputation, with surgeons attempting to preserve biological joints as much as possible.

Lower limb amputees can relearn to walk safely and comfortably within their new biomechanical

constraints by being fitted with a prosthesis. A prosthesis typically consists of a socket, fitted securely around the residual limb, a pylon, which aids in shock absorption during walking and running, and a prosthetic ankle joint and foot. Transfemoral amputees will also have a mechanical knee joint, which can be computer assisted. Osseointegration is an anchoring method in which the prosthesis is directly attached through the weight-bearing bone and is more commonly used with transfemoral amputees. Different commercially available prosthetic ankles and feet vary in the amount of energy that is stored and then returned during the pre-swing phase of the gait cycle.

Special prostheses also exist for different uses, such as sprinting. Oscar Pistorius, a bilateral transtibial amputee and Paralympics 400 m sprinter who was born with a congenital absence of the fibulas, bilaterally, runs in a pair of J-shaped carbon fibre prosthetic limbs nicknamed 'Cheetahs'. Leading up to the 2008 Olympics in Beijing, Pistorius attempted to qualify for the 400 m able-bodied race and the issue was raised of whether his prostheses gave him an unfair advantage over other able-bodied sprinters. The International Amateur Athletics Federation (IAAF) commissioned Professor Peter Bruggemann to undertake biomechanical and physiological testing on the prostheses. Compared to an able-bodied athlete running at the same speed, Professor Bruggemann reported the Cheetahs increased energy efficiency by 25%, increased energy return threefold compared with the human ankle joint and gave Pistorius a 30% greater mechanical advantage. This led the IAAF to declare the Cheetahs constituted an unfair technical advantage and banned Pistorius from the Olympics, a decision that was later overturned by the Court of Arbitration for Sport.

Lower limb amputees first practise walking and weight-bearing using a generic prosthetic device called an early walking aid (EWA). An EWA can be used as early as 1 week postoperatively and has benefits such as reduced oedema, faster healing of the residual limb and less time between surgery and casting for the functional prosthesis. An EWA consists of a rigid frame and a pneumatic sleeve, which is inflated around the residual limb. There are several types of EWAs that differ according to the level of amputation and, for transtibial amputees, movement at the knee joint (articulated versus non-articulated). Research has shown that, for transtibial amputees, there are no clear long-term benefits of walking with either an EWA that facilitates a more natural walking pattern by allowing flexion and extension at the knee joint (the Amputee Mobility Aid – AMA, Ortho Europe) or an EWA that maintains the biological knee joint in extension (the Pneumatic Post Amputation – PPAM aid, Ortho Europe). At discharge from rehabilitation, transtibial amputees who walked with either the AMA or the PPAM had improved walking performance to similar levels and did not show any differences in temporal-spatial or kinematic variables despite very different gait patterns with the EWAs during early rehabilitation (Barnett et al., 2009).

Temporal-spatial parameters

Lower limb amputees exhibit modified gait patterns and, in the case of unilateral amputation, often asymmetrical profiles between the intact and affected limbs. Transtibial and transfemoral amputees walk more slowly than age-matched, able-bodied subjects and expend more metabolic energy per unit distance walked. Transfemoral amputees often walk more slowly than transtibial amputees with walking speeds typically ranging from 1.0 to 1.3 m/s during level walking, with older, vascular amputees walking more slowly than younger, traumatic amputees. The amount of energy expenditure differs according to the level of amputation, and the mass, alignment and inertial properties of the prosthesis. Unilateral amputees spend less time in stance on their affected limb compared with their intact limb, and take longer steps with the affected limb than the intact limb.

Kinematics

Transtibial amputees have considerably reduced joint range of motion at the ankle as the prosthetic ankle/foot complex does not allow for active plantarflexion. The shape of the commonly used patellar-tendon bearing (PTB) socket may limit joint mobility of the knee, particularly knee flexion, when performing more complex tasks, such as stair descent. Transtibial and transfemoral amputees do not typically exhibit ankle plantarflexion during the transition from terminal double support to swing. Without the necessary energy generation for push-off, muscles proximal to the site of the amputation must compensate for inadequate ankle joint function. These compensations are usually provided by the hip musculature. The muscles surrounding the knee joint are

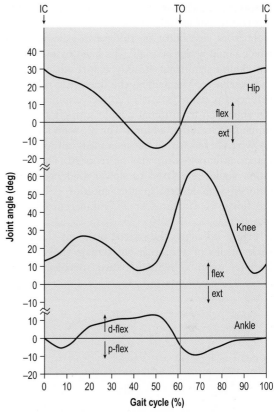

Fig. 7.6 • Sagittal plane hip, knee and ankle angles during walking in a transtibial amputation. The ankle angle shows slight abnormalities. Abbreviations as in Figure 2.5.

relatively unaffected in transtibial amputees (with the exception of gastrocnemius), however, kinematic adaptations still occur.

Figure 7.6 shows the sagittal plane hip, knee and ankle angles of a 47-year-old male transtibial amputee using a multiflex foot, walking with a cycle time of 1.26 s (cadence 95 steps/min), stride length 1.45 m and speed 1.15 m/s, all of which are towards the lower end of the normal range. The hip and knee angles are within normal limits. The ankle angle is also nearly normal, although the movement into plantarflexion in pre-swing is of relatively low magnitude and occurs a little late. This is because it is a passive movement, resulting from the removal of loading from the elastic foot mechanism, rather than the active plantarflexion seen in able-bodied subjects.

Some studies have shown that transtibial amputees lack the normal stance phase knee flexion (Powers et al., 1998; Sanderson and Martin, 1997). This could be in part due to weakness in the knee extensor muscles, which are required to contract eccentrically during this phase of the gait cycle, or feelings of instability or the prosthesis buckling, which could result in a fall. The knee extensors often exhibit significant atrophy as a result of disuse and weakness. Maintaining the knee in a relatively extended position facilitates greater stability during the transition from initial double support to single support on the affected limb. The hip joint kinematics typically fall within normal ranges, although hip extension in pre-swing may be reduced. This adaptation could be related to slower walking speeds, reduced step length, greater anterior pelvic tilt, hip flexor contractures or a combination of these factors.

Figure 7.7 shows the sagittal plane hip, knee and ankle angles of a 17-year-old female transfemoral amputee with a hydraulic knee mechanism and illustrates that transfemoral amputees exhibit virtually no stance phase-knee flexion when ambulating with non-computerised prosthetic knee joints. The amount of knee flexion in the swing phase falls within the normal range. The hip angle profile follows the normal pattern of increasing hip extension into pre-swing, followed by increasing hip flexion after toe off. However, the hip shows a sudden increase in flexion late in the swing phase when the knee mechanism reaches its extension stop and the momentum of the swinging leg is transferred to the thigh. Flexibility in the prosthetic foot leads to a fairly normal pattern of ankle motion, although the magnitudes of these movements are less than normal.

Kinetics

Examining the kinetic profiles, joint moments and powers of lower limb amputees could reveal internal adaptations that occur as a result of the amputation. Propulsive forces and impulses for the affected limb are reduced, and this is related to the absence of the power-generating plantarflexor muscles, while the braking force and impulse are not too dissimilar to the intact limb during level walking. Vertical ground reaction forces on the affected side are flattened and reduced in magnitude, and may not show the typical 'double hump' profile seen in able-bodied subjects. This could be in part due to slower walking speeds, but also an attempt to reduce loading on the residual limb/socket interface.

Internal joint moment and power profiles illustrate some compensatory adaptations related to the loss of musculature at either the transtibial or transfemoral levels. Figure 7.8 shows the sagittal plane hip, knee and ankle: (a) angles, (b) joint moments and (c) joint powers of the prosthetic leg for eight transfemoral amputee subjects who walked with two different prosthetic knees: the C-Leg® (a microprocessor-controlled knee) and Mauch SNS® (a non-computerised prosthesis) at a controlled speed of 1.11 ± 0.1 m/s and with a step length of 0.66 ± 0.04 m for the C-Leg® 0.70 ± 0.06 m for the Mauch SNS®. The hip plays an important role during pre-swing when the hip flexor muscles contract concentrically to ensure adequate foot clearance in the absence of active ankle plantarflexion. This is seen by a larger hip flexor moment and power generation burst (labelled H3) on the affected side compared with able-bodied subjects. The knee joint moments and powers during stance are typically very low or

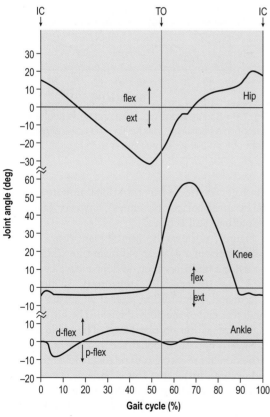

Fig. 7.7 • Sagittal plane hip, knee and ankle angles during walking in a transfemoral amputee. The main abnormality is hyperextension of the knee, from before initial contact to just before toe off. Abbreviations as in Figure 2.5.

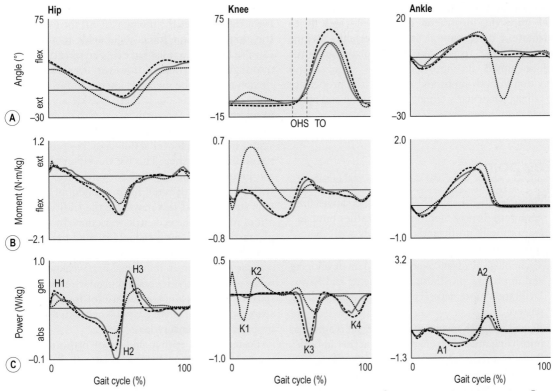

Fig. 7.8 • Kinematics and kinetics of prosthetic limb for subjects wearing C-Leg® (solid line) versus Mauch SNS® (dashed line) versus control group (dotted line) (Segal et al., 2006). For all subjects and trials, average (a) angle curves, (b) moment curves, and (c) power curves are shown for hip, knee, and ankle for controlled walking speed (1.11±0.1 m/s).

H1 = peak sagittal-plane hip power in early stance (+)
H2 = peak sagittal-plane hip power in mid-stance (−)
H3 = peak sagittal-plane hip power in late stance (+)
K1 = peak sagittal-plane knee power in early stance (−)
K2 = peak sagittal-plane knee power in mid-stance (+)
K3 = peak sagittal-plane knee power in late stance (−)
K4 = peak sagittal-plane knee power in late swing (−)
A1 = peak sagittal-plane ankle power in early stance (−)
A2 = peak sagittal-plane ankle power in late stance (+)
OHS = opposite heelstrike; TO = toe off. Positive (+) indicates power produced; negative (-) indicates power absorbed.

approach zero. By keeping the affected knee in a more extended position, the lever arm between the knee joint and the ground reaction force vector is relatively short, resulting in small knee joint moments and hence joint powers. Ankle joint moment and power profiles are arguably the most affected joint kinetic parameters because of the mechanical limitations of the prosthetic ankle–foot complex. Without active plantarflexion of the prosthetic ankle and inadequate power generation from the absent plantarflexor musculature, the ankle moment of the affected limb is substantially reduced in lower limb amputees. A small power absorption burst by the prosthesis (A1) is usually obvious and this has been attributed to the prosthetic foot absorbing energy as it deforms in dorsiflexion in mid- to terminal stance. Depending on the mechanical energy return, the ankle power generation burst in pre-swing (A2) is minimal.

Compared with able-bodied subjects, lower limb amputees display modified gait profiles but can learn to walk proficiently and safely with their prosthesis.

Technological advances are focused on developing and improving prosthetic components and fit to facilitate a more natural and comfortable walking pattern. Other recent research involving amputee gait is aimed at improving muscle strength and function in both limbs and reducing the propensity to falling, particularly among transfemoral and older, vascular amputees.

Key points

- Compared with able-bodied subjects, lower limb amputees display modified gait profiles but can learn to walk proficiently and safely with their prosthesis
- Technological advances are focused on developing and improving prosthetic components and fit to facilitate a more natural and comfortable walking pattern.
- Recent research involving amputee gait is aimed at improving muscle strength and function in both limbs and reducing the propensity to falling, particularly among transfemoral and older, vascular amputees.

Orthotic management

Plastic ankle foot orthoses have been used to manage weakness and spasticity about the ankle joint for over 40 years. However, the basic design has not changed significantly. The different design options consist of rigid, posterior leaf spring, and hinged. Other variations have been tried, including the plastic spiral ankle foot orthoses, and more recently the introduction of carbon-fibre posterior leaf spring ankle foot orthoses.

Rigid ankle foot orthoses, as the name suggests, are of a completely rigid design which aim to block all movement about the ankle joint and foot in all planes. These are usually made from moulded plastic that extend up the back of the shank and under the foot to the metatarsophalangeal joint, although sometimes this is extended over the whole length of the foot. The rigid design of the orthoses has the effect of supporting a dorsiflexion moment produced by the ground reaction force about the ankle by providing a posteriorly directed force on the anterior tibial strap, which prevents or controls tibial movement over the foot. In this way the stiffness of the rigid

ankle foot orthosis produces a plantarflexion moment that opposes the moment about the ankle from the ground reaction force. Rigid ankle foot orthoses can also be used to resist knee flexion by setting them into slight plantarflexion, however, if excessive knee flexion needs to be managed knee orthoses may give more direct control, or if there is ankle involvement using knee ankle foot orthoses may be a better option. To aid the progression of the body over the stance limb, or roll over action, a rocker profile is often added to the shoe. This has the effect of allowing the progression of the tibia forwards over the foot without necessarily requiring movement of the ankle joint itself. In fact this may have the additional benefit of reducing the eccentric work done by the ankle plantarflexors, if this is the intention of the orthosis. The clinical guidelines for the use of rigid ankle foot orthoses are when an individual has: weakness or absence of ankle dorsiflexors and plantarflexors; severe spasticity resulting in equinovarus of the foot during swing and stance phase; weak knee extensors; and proprioceptive sensory loss.

Posterior leaf spring ankle foot orthoses, sometimes referred to as flexible plastic shell orthoses, aim to provide dorsiflexion assistance during swing phase, while giving some stability for inversion/eversion of the ankle joint. The clinical guidelines for the use of posterior leaf spring ankle foot orthoses are for: weakness or absence of dorsiflexors; good pronation/supination stability; absence of foot varus or valgus; absence to moderate spasticity; and good knee stability.

Posterior leaf spring ankle foot orthoses are usually too flexible to give support in the transverse plane movement of the foot to the tibia, although this will in part depend in the 'trim lines', i.e. the width and thickness of the material of the posterior leaf spring (Fig. 7.9). The trim lines of posterior leaf spring ankle foot orthoses are critical to what these orthoses are capable of. Traditionally these have primarily been used for dorsiflexion assistance during swing phase to prevent foot drop. In this case not much material will be required to stop the foot plantarflexing as this will have to support the weight of the foot, or at most resist spastic muscle activity of the plantarflexors. However, clinically posterior leaf spring ankle foot orthoses may also be used to assist the eccentric action of plantarflexors during stance phase. This may be achieved by having wider trim lines which provide some resistance to movement into dorsiflexion and therefore improve the control of the movement over the stance limb.

Fig. 7.9 • Otto Bock moulded plastic ankle foot orthoses. Far left: rigid; middle: alternative trim lines; far right: posterior leaf spring.

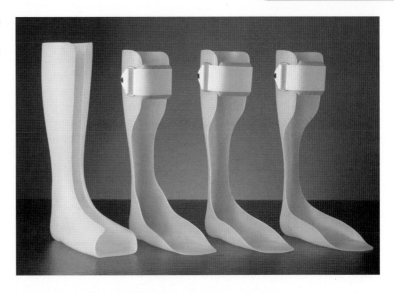

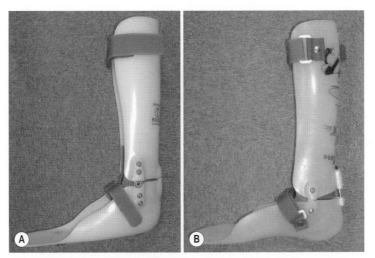

Fig. 7.10 • (A) Metal-hinged ankle foot orthoses; (B) Plastic-hinged ankle foot orthoses.

Hinged ankle foot orthoses allow free movement of the ankle in plantar flexion and dorsiflexion, but aim to block ankle movement in the coronal and transverse planes (pronation/supination and inversion/eversion). Although the movement is apparently free in the sagittal plane, the range of motion available is often controlled with plantarflexion and/or dorsiflexion stops. These plantarflexion and dorsiflexion stops are set depending on the restrictions a particular patient requires. A dorsiflexion stop may be set to stop the tibia collapsing over the foot, but yet still allowing a degree of movement of the tibia forwards over the foot. Two common hinged ankle foot orthosis designs are metal hinged (Fig. 7.10A), and plastic hinged (Fig. 7.10B). The metal hinged giving a good degree of rigidity and the plastic giving some support but not as much as the metal in the coronal and transverse planes. The plastic hinges also offer a small amount of resistance in the sagittal plane in plantarflexion and dorsiflexion. These are most often used in cerebral palsy, but may also be useful for some hemiplegic patients.

Knee ankle foot orthoses

Knee ankle foot orthoses combine the benefits of ankle foot orthoses and knee orthoses. They are generally used when larger moments are required to control the knee and when there is both substantial lack of control and stability of the ankle and knee joints. The designs of knee ankle foot orthoses can be divided into two categories, conventional and cosmetic. Conventional knee ankle foot orthoses are constructed using leather and metal, with the leather forming the straps and pads and the metal forming the side steels. Cosmetic, contemporary or plastic knee ankle foot orthoses are constructed in a similar way to plastic ankle foot orthoses with metal hinges joining the sections (Fig. 7.11). These braces are most often used in poliomyelitis, spinal cord injury, muscular dystrophy and multiple sclerosis.

Foot orthoses

Foot orthoses are shaped or moulded inserts for the shoe, which aim to hold the foot in position, change the foot position, offload a painful part of the foot or change the range of motion of either the whole foot or between the different segments of the foot. Foot orthoses can have direct effect of the segments of the foot, but they can also have significant clinical effects indirectly much further up the body to the pelvis, lower back and arguably as far up as the shoulders and neck.

Foot orthoses come in many shapes and forms, and the most basic form consist of simple ethyl vinyl acetate (EVA) wedges; some are pre-made contoured devices which may or may not need some form of modification to the patient's prescription. Lockard (1988) highlighted the fact there are many classification systems used to describe shoe inserts.

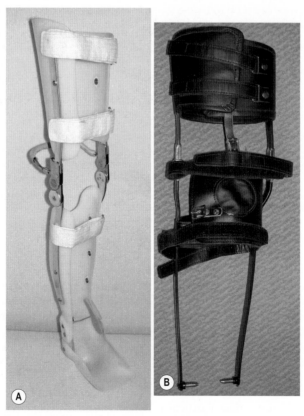

Fig. 7.11(A,B) • Knee ankle foot orthoses (KAFO): (A) cosmetic KAFO; (B) conventional KAFO.

These range from the description of the properties of the materials used, i.e. soft, semi-rigid or rigid, to the type of procedure used to construct the appliance, i.e. moulded and non-moulded. Anthony (1991) defines an orthoses as 'an orthopaedic device which is designed to promote the structural integrity of the joints of the foot and lower limb, by resisting ground reaction forces that cause abnormal skeletal motion to occur during the stance phase of gait'. Root et al. (1977) suggests they 'assist in controlling foot geometry and force direction, stabilising joints and reducing muscle contractions'.

The foot is an extremely complex system of articulating segments. Therefore the movements of the foot and ankle cannot be completely explained by rotations about a single plane but by a combination of movements in all three planes. This makes the assessment of the foot and the action of foot orthoses one of the most complex biomechanical systems in the body. This fact is compounded by the fact that the analysis of the foot, up until fairly recently, has been only considered as a single segment due to restrictions in movement analysis technology. It is highly likely that in the coming years our knowledge of foot function and the effects of foot orthotic management will be greatly expanded.

Different configurations of ankle foot orthoses can be used to block movement about the ankle joint, assist with muscle function present, or allow free movement within 'safe' limits. The use of ankle foot orthoses can have clinical effects at the ankle, knee, hip and pelvis. Foot orthoses can have a direct effect on the foot and ankle movement and the ground reaction forces, and a clinically significant effect on the control and function of the knee, hip and pelvis. The nature of each individual's muscle and joint function dictates which would be the most effective orthotic management.

Key points

- Different configurations of ankle foot orthoses can be used to block movement about the ankle joint, assist with muscle function present, or allow free movement within 'safe' limits.
- The use of ankle foot orthoses can have clinical effects at the ankle, knee, hip and pelvis.
- Foot orthoses can have a direct effect on the foot and ankle movement and the ground reaction forces, and a clinically significant effect on the control and function of the knee, hip and pelvis.
- The nature of each individual's muscle and joint function dictates which would be the most effective orthotic management.

References

Aaboe, J., Bliddal, H., Messier, S.P., et al., 2011. Effects of an intensive weight loss program on knee joint loading in obese adults with knee osteoarthritis. Osteoarthritis Cartilage 19 (7), 822–828.

Andriacchi, T.P., 1994. Dynamics of knee malalignment. Orthop. Clin. North Am. 25, 395–403.

Anthony, R.J., 1991. The manufacture and use of functional foot orthosis. Karger, Basal, Switzerland.

Baliunas, A.J., Hurwitz, D.E., Ryals, A.B., et al., 2002. Increased knee joint loads during walking are present in subjects with knee osteoarthritis. Osteoarthritis Cartilage 10, 573–579.

Barnett, C., Vanicek, N., Polman, R., et al., 2009. Kinematic gait adaptations in unilateral transtibial amputees during rehabilitation. Prosthet. Orthot. Int. 33, 141–153.

Beaulieu, M.L., Lamontagne, M., Beaule, P.E., 2010. Lower limb biomechanics during gait do not return to normal following total hip arthroplasty. Gait Posture 32, 269–273.

Bennett, D., Humphreys, L., O'Brien, S., et al., 2008. Gait kinematics of age-stratified hip replacement patients – a large scale, long-term follow-up study. Gait Posture 28, 194–200.

Briem, K., Ramsey, D.K., Newcomb, W., et al., 2007. Effects of the amount of valgus correction for medial compartment knee osteoarthritis on clinical outcome, knee kinetics and muscle co-contraction after opening wedge high tibial osteotomy. J. Orthop. Res. 25 (3), 311–318.

Butler, R.J., Marchesi, S., Royer, T., et al., 2007. The effect of a subject-specific amount of lateral wedge on knee mechanics in patients with medial knee osteoarthritis. J. Orthop. Res. 25 (9), 1121–1127.

Crenshaw, S.J., Pollo, F.E., Calton, E.F., 2000. Effect of lateral-wedged insoles on kinetics of the knee. Clin. Orthop. Relat. Res. 375, 185–192.

DeFrances, C.J., Lucas, C.A., Buie, V.C., et al., 2008. 2006 National Hospital Discharge Survey. National Center for Health Statistics, Hyattsville, MD.

Foucher, K.C., Hurwitz, D.E., Wimmer, M.A., 2007. Preoperative gait adaptations persist one year after surgery in clinically well-functioning total hip replacement patients. J. Biomech. 40, 3432–3437.

Foucher, K.C., Hurwitz, D.E., Wimmer, M.A., 2009. Relative importance of gait vs. joint positioning on hip contact forces after total hip replacement. J. Orthop. Res. 27, 1576–1582.

Goh, J.C., Bose, K., Khoo, B.C., 1993. Gait analysis study on patients with varus osteoarthrosis of the knee. Clin. Orthop. Relat. Res. 294, 223–231.

Harato, K., Nagura, T., Matsumoto, H., et al., 2010. Extension limitation in standing affects weight-bearing asymmetry after unilateral total knee arthroplasty. J. Arthroplasty 25 (2), 225–229.

Harrington, E.D., Lin, R.S., Gage, J.R., 1984. Use of the anterior floor reaction orthosis in patients with cerebral palsy. Orthotics and Prosthetics 37, 34–42.

Hewett, T.E., Noyes, F.R., Barber-Westin, S.D., et al., 1998. Decrease in knee joint pain and increase in function in patients with medial compartment arthrosis: a prospective analysis of valgus bracing. Ortopedica 21 (2), 131–138.

Hicks, R., Tashman, S., Cary, J.M., et al., 1985. Swing phase control with knee friction in juvenile amputees. J. Orthop. Res. 3, 198–201.

Hurwitz, D.E., Sumner, D.R., Andriacchi, T.P., et al., 1998. Dynamic knee loads during gait predict proximal tibial bone distribution. J. Biomech. 31 (5), 423–430.

Hurwitz, D.E., Ryals, A.B., Case, J.P., et al., 2002. The knee adduction moment during gait in subjects with knee osteoarthritis is more closely correlated with static alignment than radiographic disease severity, toe out angle and pain. J. Orthop. Res. 20, 101–107.

Jones, R.K., Nester, C.J., Kim, W.Y., et al., 2006. Direct and Indirect Orthotic Management of Medial Compartment Osteoarthritis of the Knee. ESMAC and GCMAS Meeting, Amsterdam, 25–30 September.

Kakihana, W., Akai, M., Nakazawa, K., et al., 2007. Inconsistent knee varus moment reduction caused by a lateral wedge in knee osteoarthritis. Am. J. Phys. Med. Rehabil. 86 (6), 446–454.

Keating, E.M., Faris, P.M., Ritter, M.A., et al., 1993. Use of lateral heel and sole wedges in the treatment of medial osteoarthritis of the knee. Orthop. Rev. 19, 921–924.

Kim, W.Y., Richards, J., Jones, R.K., et al., 2004. A new biomechanical model for the functional assessment of knee osteoarthritis. Knee 11 (3), 225–231.

Kirkley, A., Webster-Bogaert, S., Litchfield, R., et al., 1999. The effect of bracing on varus gonarthrosis. J. Bone Joint Surg. Am. 81, 539–548.

Kurtz, S., Ong, K., Lau, E., et al., 2007. Projections of primary and revision hip and knee arthroplasty in the United States from 2005 to 2030. J. Bone Joint Surg. Am. 89, 780–785.

Lehmann, J.F., Condon, S.M., Price, R., et al., 1987. Gait abnormalities in hemiplegia: their correction by ankle-foot orthoses. Arch. Phys. Med. Rehabil. 68, 763–771.

Lockard, M.A., 1988. Foot orthoses. Phys. Ther. 68 (12), 1866–1873.

Lindenfeld, T.N., Hewett, T.E., Andriacchi, T.P., 1997. Joint loading with valgus bracing in patients with varus gonarthrosis. Clin. Orthop. Relat. Res. 344, 290–297.

Mandeville, D., Osternig, L., Chou, L.S., 2007. The effect of total knee replacement on dynamic support of the body during walking and stair ascent. Clin. Biomech. (Bristol, Avon) 22, 787–794.

Matsumo, H., Kadowaki, K., Tsuji, H., 1997. Generation II knee bracing for severe medial compartment osteoarthritis of the knee. Arch. Phys. Med. Rehabil. 78, 745–749.

Mauer, A.C., Draganich, L.F., Pandya, N., et al., 2005. Bilateral total knee arthroplasty increases the propensity to trip on an obstacle. Clin. Orthop. Relat. Res. 433, 160–165.

McClelland, J.A., Webster, K.E., Feller, J.A., 2007. Gait analysis of patients following total knee replacement: a systematic review. Knee 14 (4), 253–263.

Messier, S.P., Loeser, R.F., Mitchell, M.N., et al., 2000. Exercise and weight loss in obese older adults with knee osteoarthritis: a preliminary study. J. Am. Geriatr. Soc. 48 (9), 1062–1072.

Messier, S.P., Gutekunst, D.J., Davis, C., et al., 2005. Weight loss reduces knee-joint loads in overweight and obese older adults with knee osteoarthritis. Arthritis Rheum. 52 (7), 2026–2032.

Miki, H., Sugano, N., Hagio, K., et al., 2004. Recovery of walking speed and symmetrical movement of the pelvis and lower extremity joints after unilateral THA. J. Biomech. 37, 443–455.

Milner, C., 2009. Is gait normal after total knee arthroplasty? Systematic review of the literature. J. Orthop. Sci. 14, 114–120.

Nankaku, M., Tsuboyama, T., Kakinoki, R., et al., 2007. Gait analysis of patients in early stages after total hip arthroplasty: effect of lateral trunk displacement on walking efficiency. J. Orthop. Sci. 12, 550–554.

Nantel, J., Termoz, N., Vendittoli, P.A., et al., 2009. Gait patterns after total hip arthroplasty and surface replacement arthroplasty. Arch. Phys. Med. Rehabil. 90, 463–469.

National Joint Registry for England and Wales, 2009. 6th Annual Report. Online: www.njrcentre.org.uk/njrcentre/AbouttheNJR/Publicationsandreports/Annualreports/tabid/86/Default.aspx (accessed xxx).

Õunpuu, S., Davis, R.B., DeLuca, P.A., 1996. Joint kinetics: methods, interpretation and treatment decision-making in children with cerebral palsy and myelomeningocele. Gait Posture 4, 62–78.

Peat, G., McCarney, R., Croft, P., 2001. Knee pain and osteoarthritis in older adults: a review of community burden and current use of primary health care. Ann. Rheum. Dis. 60, 91–97.

Perron, M., Malouin, F., Moffet, H., et al., 2000. Three-dimensional gait analysis in women with a total hip arthroplasty. Clin. Biomech. (Bristol, Avon) 15, 504–515.

Pollo, F.E., 1998. Bracing and heel wedging for unicompartmental osteoarthritis of the knee. Am. J. Knee Surg. 11 (1), 47–50.

Pollo, F.E., Otis, J.C., Backus, S.L., et al., 2002. Reduction of medial compartment loads with valgus bracing of the osteoarthritic knee. Am. J. Sports Med. 23 (6), 496–502.

Powers, C.M., Rao, S., Perry, J., 1998. Knee kinetics in trans-tibial amputee gait. Gait Posture 8, 1–7.

Prodromos, C.C., Andriacchi, T.P., Galante, J.O., 1985. A relationship between gait and clinical changes following high tibial osteotomy. J. Bone Joint Surg. Am. 67, 1188–1194.

Root, M.L., Orien, W.P., Weed, J.H., 1977. Normal and Abnormal Function of the Foot. Clin, Biomech 2.

Ranawat, A.S., Ranawat, C.S., Elkus, M., et al., 2005. Total knee arthroplasty for severe valgus deformity. J. Bone Joint Surg. Am. 87, 271–284.

Richards, J.D., Sanchez-Ballester, J., Jones, R.K., et al., 2005. A comparison of knee braces during walking for the treatment of osteoarthritis of the medial compartment of the knee. J. Bone Joint Surg. Br. 87 (7), 937–939.

Sanderson, D.J., Martin, P.E., 1997. Lower extremity kinematic and kinetic adaptations in unilateral below-knee amputees during walking. Gait Posture 6, 126–136.

Schipplein, O.D., Andriacchi, T.P., 1991. Interaction between active and passive knee stabilizers during level walking. J. Orthop. Res. 9, 113–119.

Segal, A.D., Orendurff, M.S., Klute, G.K., 2006. Kinematic and kinetic comparisons of transfemoral amputee gait using C-Leg® and Mauch SNS® prosthetic knees. J. Rehabil. Res. Dev. 43, 857–870.

Shimada, S., Kobayashi, S., Wada, M., et al., 2006. Effect of disease severity on response to lateral wedged shoe insole for medial compartment knee osteoarthritis. Arch. Phys. Med. Rehabil. 87, 1436–1451.

Tanaka, R., Shigematsu, M., Motooka, T., et al., 2010. Factors influencing the improvement of gait ability after total hip arthroplasty. J. Arthroplasty 25, 982–985.

Tashman, S., Hicks, R., Jendrzejczyk, D.J., 1985. Evaluation of a prosthetic shank with variable inertial properties. Clinical Prosthetics and Orthotics 9, 23–28.

Timoney, J., et al., 1993. Return of normal gait patterns after anterior cruciate ligament reconstruction. Am. J. Sports Med. 21 (6), 887–889.

Toda, Y., Segal, N., Kato, A., et al., 2001. Effect of a novel insole on the subtalar joint of patients with medial compartment osteoarthritis of the knee. J. Rheumatol. 28 (12), 2705–2710.

Vissers, M.M., Bussmann, J.B., Verhaar, J.A., et al., 2011. Recovery of physical functioning after total hip arthroplasty: systematic review and meta-analysis of the literature. Phys. Ther. 91, 615–629.

Winter, D.A., 1983. Energy generation and absorption at the ankle and knee during fast, natural, and slow cadences. Clin. Orthop. Relat. Res. 175, 147–154.

Winter, D.A., Sienko, S.E., 1988. Biomechanics of below-knee amputee gait. J. Biomech. 21 (5), 361–367.

Yoshida, Y., Mizner, R.L., Ramsey, D.K., et al., 2008. Examining outcomes from total knee arthroplasty and the relationship between quadriceps strength and knee function over time. Clin. Biomech. (Bristol, Avon) 23 (1), 320–328.

Zeni Jr., J.A., Snyder-Mackler, L., 2010. Most patients gain weight in the 2 years after total knee arthroplasty: comparison to a healthy control group. Osteoarthritis Cartilage 18, 510–514.

Zhang, W., Moskowitz, R.W., Nuki, G., et al., 2008. OARSI recommendations for the management of hip and knee osteoarthritis, Part II: OARSI evidence-based, expert consensus guidelines. Osteoarthritis Cartilage 16 (2), 137–162.

Index

Note: Page numbers in *italics* refer to boxes, figures and tables.